T0178030

Register Now for Online Access to Your Book!

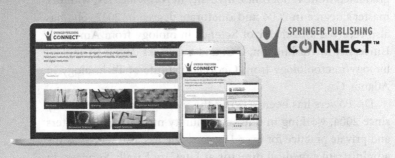

Your print purchase of *Handbook of Geropsychiatry for the Advanced Practice Nurse: Mental Healthcare for the Older Adult* **includes online access to the contents of your book—** increasing accessibility, portability, and searchability!

Access today at:
http://connect.springerpub.com/content/book/978-0-8261-5751-5
or scan the QR code at the right with your smartphone
and enter the access code below.

F2Y4TH2M

Scan here for quick access.

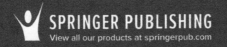

SPRINGER PUBLISHING
View all our products at springerpub.com

Leigh Powers, DNP, MSN, MS, APRN, PMHNP-BC, is a board-certified psychiatric mental health nurse practitioner. She graduated from Vanderbilt University in Nashville, TN, with her master's degree in 2004 and doctorate degree in 2012. She has also received a Bachelor of Science in biology from American University in Washington, DC, and a master's degree in applied biology/microbiology from Georgia Institute of Technology in Atlanta, GA.

Dr. Powers has been serving the mental health community since 2004, working in both community mental health centers and private practice for over 15 years. She has also served as the administrative medical director at LifeCare Family Services. In addition to her clinical practice, Dr. Powers has continued to educate future clinicians. She is currently an assistant professor at the University of North Florida, Brooks College of Health, and serves as an instructor in the Department of Psychiatry at the Edward Via College of Osteopathic Medicine (VCOM).

Marie Smith-East, PhD, DNP, PMHNP-BC, EMT-B, is a board-certified psychiatric mental health nurse practitioner. She graduated from the University of Florida with two master's degrees: one in nursing and the other in health education and behavior. She received her doctor of nursing practice degree from the University of North Florida and her PhD in nursing from the University of Central Florida. She also has a Bachelor of Science in nursing from the University of Miami in Coral Gables, FL, and a Bachelor of Science in health education and behavior with a certificate in gerontology from the University of Florida.

Dr. Smith-East has worked in community mental health, private practice, and nursing rehabilitation settings over the past several years. In education, she has been a nursing clinical instructor and facilitator, contributing to curriculum and policy development. She is currently the Director of the Psychiatric Mental Health Nurse Practitioner Program and a Clinical Assistant Professor at Duquesne University.

HANDBOOK OF GEROPSYCHIATRY FOR THE ADVANCED PRACTICE NURSE

Mental Healthcare for the Older Adult

Leigh Powers,
DNP, MSN, MS, APRN, PMHNP-BC

Marie Smith-East,
PhD, DNP, PMHNP-BC, EMT-B

Editors

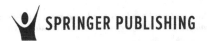 SPRINGER PUBLISHING

Springer Publishing Company, LLC
11 West 42nd Street, New York, NY 10036
www.springerpub.com
connect.springerpub.com/

Acquisitions Editor: Elizabeth Nieginski
Compositor: S4Carlisle Publishing Services

ISBN: 978-0-8261-5749-2
ebook ISBN: 978-0-8261-5751-5
DOI: 10.1891/9780826157515

20 21 22 23 24 / 5 4 3 2 1

The author and the publisher of this Work have made every effort to use sources believed to be reliable to provide information that is accurate and compatible with the standards generally accepted at the time of publication. Because medical science is continually advancing, our knowledge base continues to expand. Therefore, as new information becomes available, changes in procedures become necessary. We recommend that the reader always consult current research and specific institutional policies before performing any clinical procedure or delivering any medication. The author and publisher shall not be liable for any special, consequential, or exemplary damages resulting, in whole or in part, from the readers' use of, or reliance on, the information contained in this book. The publisher has no responsibility for the persistence or accuracy of URLs for external or third-party Internet websites referred to in this publication and does not guarantee that any content on such websites is, or will remain, accurate or appropriate.

Library of Congress Cataloging-in-Publication Data

Names: Powers, Leigh, editor. | Smith-East, Marie, editor.
Title: Handbook of geropsychiatry for the advanced practice nurse : mental healthcare for the older adult / Leigh Powers, Marie Smith-East, editors.
Description: New York : Springer Publishing Company, [2021] | Includes bibliographical references and index.
Identifiers: LCCN 2020052121 (print) | LCCN 2020052122 (ebook) | ISBN 9780826157492 (paperback) | ISBN 9780826157515 (ebook)
Subjects: MESH: Mental Disorders—nursing | Geriatric Nursing—methods | Advanced Practice Nursing—methods | Aged—psychology | Nursing Assessment—methods
Classification: LCC RC954 (print) | LCC RC954 (ebook) | NLM WY 152 | DDC 618.97/0231—dc23
LC record available at https://lccn.loc.gov/2020052121
LC ebook record available at https://lccn.loc.gov/2020052122

The ORCID for Marie Smith-East is: https://orcid.org/0000-0002-8238-4268

Contact us to receive discount rates on bulk purchases.
We can also customize our books to meet your needs.
For more information please contact: sales@springerpub.com

Printed in the United States of America.

Contents

Contents

Contributors

Abimbola Farinde, PhD, PharmD   Professor, College of
Business, Columbia Southern University, Orange Beach, Alabama

Deana Goldin, PhD, DNP, APRN, FNP-BC, PMHNP-BC
Family Nurse Practitioner Program Leader, Clinical Assistant
Professor, Florida International University, Nicole Wertheim
College of Nursing and Health Sciences, Miami, Florida

Matthew Keeslar, PA-C   Instructor of Urology, School of
Medicine, Oregon Health and Science University, Portland,
Oregon

David J. Mokler, PhD   Professor Emeritus of Pharmacology,
Department of Biomedical Sciences, College of Osteopathic
Medicine, University of New England, Biddeford, Maine

Leigh Powers, DNP, MSN, MS, APRN, PMHNP-BC   Assistant
Professor, AP Post-MSN DNP Program Director, School of
Nursing, Brooks College of Health, University of North Florida,
Jacksonville, Florida

Alan W. Skipper, DNP, APRN, FNP-BC   Assistant Professor,
School of Nursing, Georgia Southern University, Statesboro,
Georgia

Marie Smith-East, PhD, DNP, PMHNP-BC, EMT-B   Clinical
Assistant Professor, Director of the Psychiatric Mental Health
Nurse Practitioner Program, School of Nursing, Duquesne
University, Pittsburgh, Pennsylvania

William S. Sutton, DNP, APRN, CRNP-PMH   Psychiatric
Mental Health Nurse Practitioner, Kraus Behavioral Health,
Catonsville, Maryland

Contributors

Helene Vossos, DNP, MSN, APRN, ANP-BC, PMHNP-BC
Assistant Professor of Nursing, Director of PMHNP-DNP
Program, Brooks College of Health, University of North Florida,
Jacksonville, Florida

Joanne Zanetos, DNP, MSN   Assistant Professor, School
of Nursing, Waters College of Health Professions, Georgia
Southern University, Statesboro, Georgia

Chapter Reviewers

Barbara K. Bailes, EdD, RN, ANP-BC   Associate Professor, Cizik School of Nursing, The University of Texas, Austin, Texas

Abimbola Farinde, PhD, PharmD   Professor, College of Business, Columbia Southern University, Orange Beach, Alabama

David J. Mokler, PhD   Professor Emeritus of Pharmacology, Department of Biomedical Sciences, College of Osteopathic Medicine, University of New England, Armidale, Australia

Rebecca Perez, BSN, RN, CCM   CMSA Director of Product Development and Education, CMSA Foundation Executive Director, Fraser Imagineers, Little Rock, Arkansas

Susan Wehry, MD   Chief of Geriatrics, Department of Primary Care, College of Osteopathic Medicine (UNE COM), University of New England, Biddeford, Maine

Preface

The ability to reduce the psychological burden of illness among older adults is necessary as individuals are living longer and experiencing decreases in function that are often associated with age-related conditions (National Institute on Aging, 2020). Advanced practice nurses are skilled in relieving the burden of illness among older adults through specialized training and providing treatment in a variety of clinical settings. While geriatric-focused psychiatric content exists, advanced practice nurses can benefit from specialized clinical pearls and insights specific for the advanced practice nurse providing holistic mental healthcare.

This handbook offers advanced practice nurses, nurse educators, and graduate nursing students a reference that is intended to be supplemental to uniquely providing care for older adults, which includes an overview of the aging process as well as assessing and developing treatment plans for older adults with mental health disorders. As older adults often work collaboratively with family, friends, caregivers, and healthcare providers, approaches to such relationships are explored and further developed in order to serve as an additional resource for providing mental healthcare that can contribute to the overall success of treatment.

The text provides an interprofessional box that encourages and assists the advanced practice nurse navigating through interdisciplinary collaborative practice. Such interprofessional partnerships can enhance care—particularly in cases of complexity. Advanced practice nurses can utilize the provided case studies to identify and modify service delivery that promotes evidence-based practice.

REFERENCE

National Institute on Aging. (2020). *Strategic directions for research 2020–2025*. Retrieved from https://www.nia.nih.gov/sites/default/files/2020-05/nia-strategic-directions-2020-2025.pdf

DISCLOSURES

Leigh Powers, DNP, MSN, MS, APRN, PMHNP-BC, reports no conflicting interests.

Marie Smith-East, PhD, DNP, PMHNP-BC, EMT-B, reports no conflicting interests.

CHAPTER 1

BASIC FOUNDATIONS OF AGING

LEIGH POWERS

LEARNING OBJECTIVES

After reviewing this chapter, practitioners will be able to:

- define aging, longevity, and life expectancy
- recognize factors that may impact longevity
- summarize major normal age-related physiological and psychosocial changes in humans
- explain domains that may promote healthy aging
- discuss the importance of the annual wellness visit in supporting healthy aging

■ INTRODUCTION

According to *Guinness World Records*, the current oldest living individual as of 2019 is 116 years old, with the longest living individual recorded to be 122 years and 164 days old (Guinness World Records, 2019). In the United States, the National Center for Health Statistics has determined the average life expectancy to be 78.6 years for all races, with 76.1 for males and 81.1 for females (Murphy et al., 2018). The top ten leading causes of death in the United States currently are heart disease, cancer, unintentional injuries, chronic lower respiratory diseases, stroke, Alzheimer's disease, diabetes, influenza and pneumonia, kidney disease, and suicide, respectively (Murphy et al., 2017).

Definitions of aging continue to evolve. In this chapter, aging is considered a part of normal life processes that consists of the acquisition of knowledge and skills over time, the honing and maximizing of these traits, and eventually the time period in which all body systems decline from maximal functioning capacity. Normal aging processes will be reviewed in addition to factors that can affect life longevity such as genetic and environmental factors and the human response to environmental stressors. A brief review of healthy aging and holistic measures will also be discussed. Specific neurological and brain changes will be reviewed in depth in Chapter 9.

■ NORMAL AGING

Longevity describes the length of a human being's life. Numerous factors influence longevity and account for the variability in aging we see in individuals over time. Longevity can be altered through genetic and environmental factors as well as lifestyle choices. In the last 200 years, significant changes in environmental influences to longevity occurred, resulting in a substantial extension in life span. Food sources became more abundant. Scientific knowledge expanded with important discoveries in medicine and disease treatment and prevention. Living conditions overall improved with better housing options and developments in water and utility resources. All of these changes resulted in decreased premature deaths, decreased infant mortality rates, and increased survival into older age (National Institutes of Health, 2018).

Genetics may play a part in determining which individuals live past the norm into their 90s and 100s. Variations have been found in some common genes such as *APOE, FOXO3*, and *CETP* (Sebastiani et al., 2017) that may contribute to longer life spans as well as some newer gene variants recently discovered that may have protectant factors that decrease cellular damage from free radicals or decrease chromosomal errors. Currently, scientific evidence suggests the strongest influences for longevity in the first 70 to 80 years are lifestyle factors rather than genetic (National Institutes of Health, 2019).

Healthy aging is described by the World Health Organization "as the process of *developing* [emphasis added] and maintaining the functional ability that enables wellbeing in older age" (World Health Organization, 2019). Factors that can impact an individual's healthy aging include level of physical fitness, smoking/tobacco habits, alcohol use, dietary habits, stress response, and individual resilience (Figure 1.1). Responses to environmental stressors and health risks can decrease longevity by increasing disease progression and a more rapid decline in an individual's functioning level.

What is important for the practitioner to remember is that changes in one organ system do not predict decline in others and that both intra-individual and inter-individual variability are significant.

Areas of change to the body in normal aging include:

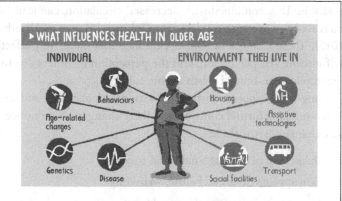

FIGURE 1.1 What influences healthy aging?

SOURCE: World Health Organization. (2019). *What is healthy ageing?* https://www.who.int/ageing/events/world-report-2015 -launch/healthy-ageing-infographic.jpg?ua=1

- integumentary
- cardiovascular
- respiratory
- genitourinary
- endocrine
- musculoskeletal
- visual/ocular
- hearing

What may be of greatest significance are changes in the ability to maintain homeostasis, a change described as homeostenosis.

Integumentary

Initially, most individuals describe aging by what changes in visual appearance, primarily the integumentary system including skin and hair as well as the connective tissues in the skin. With aging, the skin thins and becomes more susceptible to bruising and pressure sores. In addition, as the skin thins, less insulation is available. This, combined with decreased circulation, can lead to increased temperature intolerances (Johnson Memorial Health, 2015). These changes in skin appearance may negatively affect self-esteem, self-perception, and the perception by others due to the implicit bias toward youth in this culture.

Long-term exposure to the sun, chronic alcohol use, and tobacco smoking further contribute to these changes. Other noticeable changes may include:

- thickening of the fingernails and toenails
- skin appears drier and brittle, wrinkling
- loss of hair on body surface and head
- changes in pigmentation of hair leading to gray or white hair
- increased pigmentation that appear as "age spots"
- increased vulnerability to infections due to thinning of the epidermal layer

Cardiovascular

With age, the heart begins to stiffen and weaken. The valves over time become thicker and may result in an auscultated heart murmur (US National Library of Medicine, 2020). The blood vessels also lose their elasticity and may have fatty deposits build up along the walls, leading to a hardening of the vessels. This arteriosclerosis can increase the workload for the heart to continuously circulate blood (Johnson Memorial Health, 2015). With normal aging, fluid levels decrease and may reduce the overall blood volume (US National Library of Medicine, 2020). Red blood cell turnover slows, which may lead to a decreased response time to blood loss. In addition, the SA node may lose cell volume over time, slowing the heart rate.

Common cardiovascular changes in older adults may include:

- hypertension: The aorta may become thicker with less flexible muscle tissue.
- orthostatic hypotension: The baroreceptors that monitor blood pressure and assist in the maintenance of stable pressures may become less sensitive over time (US National Library of Medicine, 2020).
- congestive heart failure
- angina or chest pain: There is perceived pain when reduced blood flow to the heart occurs.
- arrhythmias

Respiratory

With aging, the airway and tissues of the respiratory system become more rigid and less malleable. The elasticity of alveoli in the lungs is decreased, creating a decreased surface area for gas exchange (American Lung Association, 2018). In addition, lung capacity may change due to the changing physiology of the chest cavity from possible osteoporosis. The muscles required for the work of breathing, the diaphragm and abdominal muscles, may be lessened, making breathing more laborious. There may be more stiffness in the chest wall, with age creating a reduced forced expiratory volume and reduced maximal oxygen consumption (Sharma & Goodwin, 2006).

These respiratory changes may lead to:

- increased susceptibility to lung infections such as pneumonia and viral infections
- increased fibrous tissue in lungs
- reduced gas exchange
- decreased ability to maintain lung capacity with increased exertion

Genitourinary

With aging, kidney function also declines. The efficiency of waste removal declines due to a decrease in kidney mass with time. The total glomeruli per kidney decreases by 300,000 from under 40 years old to the approximate age of 65 (Boss & Seegmiller, 1981). Bladder capacity decreases as we age. In younger persons, the average bladder capacity is around 500 mL to 600 mL. Over 65 years of age, the capacity is reduced to approximately 250 mL (Boss & Seegmiller, 1981). The sensation to void usually occurs when the bladder reaches half full in younger adults, but in the geriatric population this sensation may be dulled or occur much later leading the urinary incontinence. In males, by the age of 80, it is common for a majority to experience symptoms of prostatic hyperplasia resulting in obstruction and/or urinary retention (Johnson Memorial Health, 2015).

Endocrine

The endocrine system is primarily associated with hormone production and homeostasis within the body. With aging, secretion of hormones decreases overall, which can lead to increased difficulty with sleep, decreased metabolism, decreased bone mass, and changes in blood glucose regulation (Knight & Nigam, 2017). Regular exercise and decreased body fat composition can assist in counteracting some of the age-related changes.

Endocrine changes that may result with age include:

- somatopause: Decreased production of somatotropin may lead to decreased lean body mass and increased adipose tissue, such as abdominal fat, and reduced bone mass and density (Gentili & Adler, 2020).

- pineal gland calcification: Decreased secretion of melatonin can lead to sleep disturbances. It has been reported that older individuals may have 80% less melatonin than younger individuals (Knight & Nigam, 2017).

- thyroid hormone: Decreases in thyroid-stimulating hormone and triiodothyronine (T3) may contribute to decreased metabolism and weight gain (Peeters, 2008).

- insulin: Aging decreases cell sensitivity to insulin, which can increase the risk of developing type 2 diabetes (Kirkman et al., 2012).

Musculoskeletal

As the body ages, muscle mass tends to decrease and bone loss occurs. Muscles atrophy both from reduced physical activity as we age as well as reduction in protein synthesis and the number of muscle fibers. With reduced mass and strength, the muscles are unable to support the previous levels of physical strength. The contraction force and speed are reduced resulting in "senile sarcopenia" (Papa et al., 2017). Similar to the muscles, bones also shrink in their size and density, which may lead to osteoporosis, fractures, and falls. In aging, osteoclasts continue to absorb bone to release the needed calcium back into the body; however, with less physical activity the body's osteoblasts decrease deposition of new bone (Nigam et al., 2009).

Visual/Ocular

As the eye ages, the eye lens will decrease in elasticity. Cataracts can develop causing blind or foggy fields of vision. With fewer fat deposits in the pre-orbital space and eyelid, ptosis (drooping of the eyelid) can impede vision. Vision loss and blindness are quite common in the older adult population with possible contributing factors of cataracts, age-related macular degeneration, and glaucoma (National Institutes of Health, 2019). Glaucoma affects the eye's optic nerve and may lead to vision changes due to pressure changes in the eye. Cataracts form slowly over the lens of the eye and may cause partial or full vision impediments (American Optometric Association, n.d.). It may become more difficult to drive at night, as there is a diminished tolerance of glare.

Common vision/eye complaints in older adults include:

- dry eye from decreased tear production by the tear glands
- presbyopia: increased difficulty seeing objects up close
- decreased color differentiation

Hearing

One of the most common changes from aging in geriatric patients is the loss of hearing. The age-related loss of hearing is termed *presbycusis* and generally occurs gradually over time. Hearing loss is as common as one in three in the United States for individuals aged 65 to 74 and as common as one in two for those older than 75 (National Institutes of Health, 2018; National Institute on Deafness and Other Communication Disorders, 2018; Table 1.1).

In general, hearing loss occurs bilaterally and can affect an individual's ability to adapt to their surroundings and to interact with others. This can lead to confusion, anxiety, and depression due to frustration and a sense of isolation. Hearing loss can occur from numerous factors other than normal aging, including long-term exposure to environmental noises that damage the sensory hair cells (noise-induced hearing loss). Medical conditions that adversely affect hearing can include diabetes, hypertension, and some medications (National Institutes of Health, 2018). In aging, it is reported that the most common cause other than environmental and medical is the change in the inner and middle ear. The inner ear can lose elasticity and conductive properties. Speech may seem distorted due to poor quality of amplification.

Common signs of hearing loss may include:

- a ringing or buzzing in the ears
- turning up the volume on the TV or radio
- confusing similar sounding words in conversations
- watching speakers mouths for words
- having difficulty hearing conversations in rooms with moderate ambient noise levels
- thinking others mumble frequently

TABLE 1.1
Hearing Handicap Inventory Screening Questionnaire for Adults

Answer No, Sometimes, or Yes for each question.
DO NOT SKIP a question if you avoid a situation because of a hearing problem.
Does a hearing problem cause you to feel embarrassed when you meet new people?
1. Does a hearing problem cause you to feel frustrated when talking to members of your family?
2. Do you have difficulty hearing/understanding co-workers, clients, or customers?
3. Do you feel handicapped by a hearing problem?
4. Does a hearing problem cause you difficulty when visiting friends, relatives, or neighbors?
5. Does a hearing problem cause you difficulty in the movies or in the theater?
6. Does a hearing problem cause you to have arguments with family members?
7. Does a hearing problem cause you difficulty when listening to TV or radio?
8. Do you feel that any difficulty with your hearing limits or hampers your personal or social life?
9. Does a hearing problem cause you difficulty when in a restaurant with relatives or friends?

Source: Adapted from Newman, C. W., Weinstein, B. E., Jacobson, G. P., & Hug, G. A. (1990). The hearing handicap inventory for adults: Psychometric adequacy and audiometric correlates. *Ear and Hearing, 11,* 430–433. https://doi.org/10.1097/00003446-199012000-00004

CASE 1.1

Mrs. Wynonna Carroll is a 76-year-old Caucasian female who presents to an outpatient clinic with complaints of "my husband tells me I turn the television up too loud at night." This has caused an increase in arguments between the two, who have been married for 55 years. During one of these arguments, her husband suggested "that I need to see someone about my bossiness and possibly my ears." During the assessment, she occasionally asks provider to repeat questions, turning her left ear toward the provider. She reports overall her mood is "fair to middling," and denies any difficulty with persistent low mood or anxiety. She indicates that she has some occasional "aches and pains" in her left shoulder, primarily in the afternoons after waking from her daily nap, that keep her from her gardening. She indicates that she still enjoys her weekly get-togethers with her gardening group at the local YMCA and attends religious services every Saturday evening with her husband. Her energy level is good, and she remains motivated to engage in her usual activities. She talks about excitement regarding an upcoming high school reunion back home in Utah, although she does not care for the colder winters there compared to current winter climates in south Florida where she now resides in a senior residential community.

Overall, she states that she generally has a "good disposition, just when he gets on my nerves about the TV volume, I can get a bit irritated." She indicates they tend to get along most other times, but finds in the evenings when her husband gets back from golf and she wants to watch her shows, they tend to be short-tempered with one another. She denies any aggressive or assaultive behaviors on either part and states they may raise their voices, but are not verbally abusive of one another. She denies any use of substances and denies any history of psychosis or current auditory/visual hallucinations, perceptual disturbance, or delusions.

She indicates that she doesn't sleep well at night due to her husband's snoring, which wakes her between four and six times per night. She also tends to get up once during the night

(continued)

to urinate. She denies any urgency, pain, or hesitancy with urinating. She has a mild lisp when speaking and occasionally flicks her top denture out of place but is seemingly unaware of this. She denies any problems with her dentures and states she has both top and bottom dentures.

She currently takes lisinopril, calcium, a vitamin D supplement, and ibuprofen as needed for previously diagnosed hypertension, osteoporosis, and vitamin D insufficiency. She takes ibuprofen for occasional pain. She has had her wisdom teeth removed, and she had a tubal ligation after giving birth to two sons and one daughter. She scores a 28 on the MMSE and denies any significant problems with short-term memory or long-term memory, although she cannot recall exactly how long ago she last had a complete physical. In addition, provider completed a Mini-Cog assessment where she scored a 5, and a SLUMS assessment where she scored a 27. She reports no past treatment for mental illness, but then reports she did receive marital counseling in her 30s with her husband after "he went and did something foolish." She felt the counseling was beneficial at the time stating "since we're still together."

Vitals are as follows:

Height—66"

Weight—187 lbs

Blood pressure—138/88 mmHg (millimeters of mercury)

Pulse—78 bpm (beats per minute)

Respiratory rate—16 BPM or breaths per minute

Questions:

1. Based on the limited patient history and current symptoms presented so far, what else might you want to ascertain about her history and symptoms? What other specific questions might you consider related to the patient's chief complaint?

2. What referrals would you make, if any (mental health and physical health)?

Interprofessional Box

When evaluating Mrs. Carroll, you administer the MMSE as well as a PHQ-9. She receives a score of 28/30 on the MMSE and is oriented and well aware of current situations. She is pleasant and attends to the examination appropriately. She scores a 2 on the PHQ-9, with primary complaints of several nights of poor sleep and mild fatigue on less than half the days of the week. She denies any difficulty overall with persistent depression or anxiety and appears to primarily present with relationship/interpersonal problems and a possible hearing loss in her right ear. It is determined with patient request that a referral to marital therapy may be beneficial to improve communication as well as a referral to an audiologist for hearing testing or an ENT specialist. She may also benefit from a referral to physical therapy to assist with range of motion and to address her mild pain in the afternoons that keep her from gardening. A referral should also be made to dental to assist with possible adjustment of her upper dentures.

Evidence-Based Practice Box

Evidence-based practice for healthy aging focuses on disease prevention and health promotion to maintain or improve the quality of life for older adults. Programs often focus on the triad of the older adult patient, the caregiver, and the health professional, although it should be noted that many older adults do not have caregivers. Healthy aging includes chronic disease management, encouraging appropriate levels of continued exercise, and healthy eating habits. Programs for fall prevention and appropriate pain management have been implemented with success. The AARP Foundation has implemented funding to assist with the identification of late-life depression (AARP, 2019). The Robert Wood Johnson Foundation (RWJF, 2018) has supported programming on chronic disease management.

REFERENCES

American Association of Retired Persons. (2019). *AARP Foundation.* https://aarp.org/aarp-foundation/

American Lung Association. (2018, April 24). *Your aging lungs.* https://www.lung.org/blog/your-aging-lungs

American Optometric Association. (n.d.) Cataracts. https://www.aoa.org/healthy-eyes/eye-and-vision-conditions/cataract?sso=y

Boss, G. R. & Seegmiller, J. E. (1981, Dec). Age-related physiological changes and their clinical significance. *West J Med,* 135(6), 434–440.

Gentili, A. & Adler, R. (2020, April 14). What is hyposomatotropism of aging (somatopause)? *Medscape.* https://www.medscape.com/answers/126999-198980/what-is-hyposomatotropism-of-aging-somatopause#:~:text=This%20decline%20in%20the%20secretory,muscle%20mass%2C%20and%20physical%20function.

Guinness World Records. (2019, March 9). *World's oldest person confirmed as 116-year-old Kane Tanaka from Japan.* https://www.guinnessworldrecords.com/news/2019/3/worlds-oldest-person-confirmed-as-116-year-old-kane-tanaka-from-japan

Johnson Memorial Health. (2015, September 22). 9 *Physical Changes that Come With Aging.* http://blog.johnsonmemorial.org/9-physical-changes-that-come-with-aging

Kirkman, M. Sue, Briscoe, V., Clark, N., Florez, H., Hass, L. Halter, J., Huang, E., Korytkowski, M., Munshi, M., Odegard, P., Pratley, R., & Swift, C. (2012, December). Diabetes in older adults. *Diabetes Care,* 35, 2650–2664.

Knight J., Nigam Y. (2017). Anatomy and physiology of ageing 7: the endocrine system. *Nursing Times* [online], 113(8), 48–51.

Murphy, S. L., Xu, J. Q., Kochanek, K. D., & Arias, E. (2018). *Mortality in the United States, 2017* (NCHS Data Brief, No. 328). U.S. Department of Health and Human Services.

National Eye Institute. (2019). *Vision and aging resources.* https://www.nei.nih.gov/agingeye

National Institute on Deafness and Other Communication Disorders. (2018, July 17). Age-Related Hearing Loss. https://www.nidcd.nih.gov/health/age-related-hearing-loss

National Institutes of Health. (2018). *Turning discovery into health.* https://www.nih.gov/sites/default/files/about-nih/impact/impact-our-health.pdf

Nigam Y. et al. (2009) Effects of bedrest 3: musculoskeletal and immune systems, and skin. *Nursing Times, 105,* 23. https://www.nursingtimes.net/clinical-archive/orthopaedics/effects-of-bedrest-3-musculoskeletal-and-immune-systems-skin-and-self-perception-29-06-2009/

Papa EV et al. (2017). Skeletal muscle function deficits in the elderly: current perspectives on resistance training. *Journal of Nature and Science, 3*(1), e272.

Peeters, R. (2008). Thyroid hormones and aging. *Hormones, 7*(1), 28–35. doi:10.14310/horm.2002.1111035.

Robert Wood Johnson Foundation. (2018). *Our focus areas.* https://www.rwjf.org/en/our-focus-areas.html

Sebastiani, P., Gurinovich, A., Bae, H., Andersen, S., Malovini, A., Atzmon, G., Villa, F., Kraja, A. T., Ben-Avraham, D., Barzilai, N., Puca, A., & Perls, T. T. (2017, October 12). Four genome-wide association studies identify new extreme longevity variants. *Journals of Gerontology. Series A, Biological Sciences and Medical Sciences, 72*(11), 1453–1464. https://doi.org/10.1093/gerona/glx027

Sharma, G. & Goodwin, J. (2006). Effect of aging on respiratory system physiology and immunology. *Clin Interv Aging. 1*(3), 253–260.

US National Library of Medicine. (2020, October 8). *Aging changes in the heart and blood vessels.* https://medlineplus.gov/ency/article/004006.htm

WebMD Medical Reference. (2018). *Eye problems: What to expect as you age.* https://www.webmd.com/eye-health/vision-problems-aging-adults

World Health Organization. (2019). *What is healthy ageing?* https://www.who.int/ageing/healthy-ageing/en/

CHAPTER 2

THE PSYCHIATRIC EXAM IN GEROPSYCHIATRY

LEIGH POWERS

LEARNING OBJECTIVES

After reviewing this chapter, practitioners will be able to:

- identify the essential components of an initial psychiatric evaluation

- discuss unique components and requirements of an initial evaluation with geriatric mental health patients

- evaluate the results/outcome from the completion of an initial psychiatric exam to formulate an appropriate plan of treatment

■ INTRODUCTION

In this chapter, practitioners will be introduced to the psychiatric evaluation, in general, and specifically for geriatric mental health patients. Practitioners will learn about the essential components of an initial evaluation and review some of the basic methods for assessment such as rating scales and standardized assessment tools. Although a few examples will be provided within this chapter, more specific assessment tools will be reviewed for individual psychiatric disorders within the associated chapters. Common factors that practitioners may be uniquely confronted within a geriatric psychiatric evaluation will be considered.

■ THE PSYCHIATRIC EVALUATION

The psychiatric evaluation is an overall assessment of a patient's past and present status from a holistic standpoint; it reviews family dynamics, medical health, psychiatric health, impacts of trauma, social history, education, and growth/development. Evaluations may be completed in diverse settings for the geriatric population including assisted living facilities, nursing homes, patient's or family member's homes, outpatient offices, or hospitals, to name a few.

At the beginning, an initial evaluation should provide details regarding the setting, participants present, status of legal guardianship, and specific issues related to competency, reliability, and consent. Details should be provided regarding the availability of collaborative information. It has been studied and determined that often geriatric patients may present with symptoms that may vary from the classic diagnostic criteria, as it is common in this population group to minimize symptomology. Geriatric patients may also have significant comorbid complex medical illnesses that can cloud the diagnostic process or increase the difficulty of differentiating symptoms back to their etiology. It is important to ascertain their hearing status and obtain proper assistive devices as needed.

Common confounding and unique issues present during an initial psychiatric evaluation with geriatric patients should be appropriately documented. The initial evaluation may follow a general outline (Table 2.1).

This outline is to provide a template for proceeding through the evaluation but should not serve as a final agenda for all evaluations. The process should be tailored to the individual and symptoms present and abilities of the geriatric patients' recall/response participation as well as comorbid medical issues.

> **Chief Complaint**—This should provide a personalized statement of why the patient is present for an initial evaluation. Even if the patient is not aware of the reason to attend, this should be documented to provide current status of patient's understanding and

TABLE 2.1
Basic Psychiatric Evaluation Overview—Template for Assessment

Chief Complaint
■ Reason for visit in patient's own words in quotes
■ Onset of symptoms
■ Precipitating factors
History of Present Illness
■ Symptom review
■ Past psychiatric history
■ Substance use assessment
■ Social history
■ Family psychiatric and medical history
■ Medical history
■ Pain scale
Mental Status Exam
Assessment of Patient Functional Abilities
Assessment of Patient Cognitive Abilities
Plan of Treatment
■ Review of appropriate records and collaborative input
■ Review of past legal records, labs, and prescription monitoring program
■ Referrals and interprofessional collaborative care
■ Working diagnoses
■ Nonpharmacological treatment
■ Pharmacological treatment
■ Safety plan and crisis plan
■ Return for follow-up appointment

awareness. The chief complaint should be recorded in quotes. Examples include "my son is worried that I am crying too much, and I am not eating like he wants me to," or "those beetles that crawl on my face at night are getting to be too much."

History of Present Illness (HPI)—This section addresses recent or precipitating events/factors leading to the patient presenting for the initial evaluation with the associated chief complaint. The HPI should also include a psychiatric timeline of onset, magnitude, and duration of past psychiatric symptoms. The provider should use the narrative to build the case for differential and initial diagnoses by reviewing current symptoms that may align with criteria for specific diagnoses found in the *Diagnostic and Statistical Manual of Mental Disorders,* Fifth Edition (American Psychiatric Association, 2013). However, it is imperative for the provider to be aware that it is not uncommon for geriatric patients to present with less classic, alternative constellation of symptoms as well as symptoms normalized due to aging. Subjective and objectives details should be documented in addition to any collaborative statements from family members or staff present with the patient. Family member input is essential when any major neurocognitive disorder is suspected. Additional supportive documentation, such as rating scales, may be included and completed with the patient to provide supportive symptom details meeting criteria for specific diagnoses. Rating scales specific to each mental health diagnosis will be reviewed in future chapters.

Past Psychiatric History—In this section, past treatment should be reviewed. This may include:

- past treatment providers,
- length of time in past outpatient treatment,
- periods without treatment,
- types of treatment (i.e., medication management, supportive therapy, ECT, case management, intensive outpatient, etc.)
- history of inpatient psychiatric admissions (number, dates)
- past suicide and/or homicide attempts
- past self-injurious behaviors

- past known psychiatric diagnoses
- past psychotropic medication trials (success and failures)

Family History—Both medical and psychiatric family history should be documented. For geriatric patients, a majority of their parents will be deceased. Understanding familial history of past medical illnesses and deaths may provide guidance regarding the patient's current complaints. Family psychiatric history may provide red flags for the patient's diagnosis or indicate possible needs to further genetic testing.

Medical and Surgical History—Documentation should include all past and current medical diagnoses and date of onset if known. In the geriatric population, there is often a high correlation between medical complications and psychiatric illness. There is evidence that some medical disorders may serve as triggers for psychiatric disorders.

Pain Level Using Pain Scale—Although it is not a psychiatric symptom, pain can adversely affect psychiatric symptoms such as anxiety, depression, and sleep. It can be advantageous to obtain a score using a pain scale of 1 to 10 to assist in quantifying the subjective symptom. If patients are unable to verbalize or provide a numerical value to their pain, providers may find using the Wong-Baker Facial Pain Rating Scale to be of benefit (Wong Baker Faces Foundation, 2016).

Current Medical Medications and Medical Allergies—This information is a vital component of the initial evaluation, especially with geriatric patients. Due to general decreased kidney and liver functioning as well as the potential for drug–drug interactions from frequent prescribing of multiple medications, it is imperative for the practitioner to document all medications the patient is prescribed.

> **Assessment of Patient's Functional Abilities**—It is pertinent to assess a patient's current functional status. Patients should be assessed regarding their ability to complete their activities of daily living independently in two spheres—activities of daily living and instrumental daily activities (Lawton & Brody, 1969). This

information will assist the provider in formulating plans of care, interprofessional collaboration, and referrals for supportive services. This will also serve as a baseline from which the provider may later assess improvements or decline.

Mental Status Exam—A mental status exam provides a snapshot of the patient during the evaluation. This exam is not formally "given" to the patient but completed primarily through observation of the patient throughout the evaluation. Each evaluation should include reference to the patient's current mental state and be appropriately documented with relevant narrative statements (Table 2.2).

Assessment of Patient Cognitive Functioning—This is a vital component of a psychiatric evaluation for a geriatric patient. It is imperative to understand the cognitive

TABLE 2.2
Example Mental Status Review

Level of consciousness: alert, oriented, and grossly intact
Behavior: cooperative; no guarding noted
Appearance: as stated age; groomed, dressed casually, and appropriate to weather and circumstances
Mood: depressed
Affect: mood congruent, withdrawn
Speech: WNL for pt; normal tone, prosody, and volume
Thoughts: goal-directed
Memory/Attention/Concentration: intact; no apparent deficits noted
Cognitive Function: within normal limits
Insight: good
Judgment: good
Psychomotor: no psychomotor agitation or retardation noted
No reports of current or recent SIB.
No current SI/HI, intent, or plan. No reports of a/v hallucinations, perceptual disturbances, delusions, or paranoia.

A/V - auditory/visual hallucinations; SIB - self-injurious behaviors; SI/HI - suicidal ideation/homicidal ideation; WNL - within normal limits.

functioning level of a patient to formulate an accurate diagnosis and treatment. A formal assessment of cognitive functional status will include review of a patient's attention, concentration, language reception and expression, orientation, memory, and engagement. Generally, patients are given the Folstein (or Mini-Mental State Exam), which is a 30-question exam that briefly assesses cognitive impairment, often serving as an initial evaluation for major neurocognitive disorders (Folstein et al., 1975).

CASE 2.1 INITIAL EVALUATION FOR DEPRESSION AND ANXIETY

An 82-year-old woman, Mrs. S, presents with a chief complaint of anxiety and depression. "I'm so sorry to be a bother, but I just can't stop crying."

History Available

No previous mental health issues prior to age 26 when she experienced her first depressive episode. This episode included symptoms of depressed mood, loss of appetite, amotivation, and anhedonia, but no complaints of anxiety. She was treated at the time with an antidepressant, Prozac, and symptoms remitted within several months. She subsequently stopped the Prozac without any complications or reoccurrence of symptoms.

A second episode occurred around age 48 following the sudden death of one of her sons from a motor vehicle accident (MVA). It was unclear at the time whether she was experiencing a second depressive episode or a prolonged bereavement period. She was not treated at the time with medications, but did see a therapist for a few sessions, and recovered months later.

At this time, Mrs. S lives alone in an apartment in Philadelphia, PA. Her husband died suddenly 2.5 years ago from a heart attack. Her remaining two children both live out of state. Both of her sons maintain bi-weekly phone contact

(*continued*)

with the patient and visit usually once per year. She had been doing relatively well up until about 5 weeks ago when she fell in her apartment and sustained bruises but did not require hospitalization. Since then, she has been preoccupied with her failing eyesight and decreased ambulation. One son, who accompanied her to today's visit, indicates she began calling him and his brother multiple times per week, sometimes multiple times per day, with worry and being tearful. She has not been leaving the apartment as often to go shopping. She states that she does not enjoy going out anymore and feels "very sad and teary." She minimizes her decreased socialization and daily activities stating that since it is just her now, she does not need to shop as much, and she is not as hungry as she used to be. "I'm getting too old to cook for one person only." She has not been sleeping well, is unable to stop thinking at night about her health, and feels lonely, stating she is sleeping 3 to 4 hours and does not feel rested upon waking. She is not napping during the daytime. Mrs. S's son indicates they took her to her primary care provider (PCP), where she was prescribed Xanax 0.5 mg BID and Risperdal 0.5 mg qhs, but they do not feel it is helping her at this time.

Subjective

She walks into the office with a shuffling gait, masked facies, rigidity, and a tremor. She is parsimonious in her speech and her affect appears flat and apathetic; however, she complains of significant anxiety and depressed mood. She is not suicidal and appears to be globally oriented. She complains of anhedonia, anergia, amotivation, and problems with initial insomnia due to ruminating thoughts.

Questions:

1. Based upon the limited patient history and current symptoms presented so far, how do you think you might proceed with assessment/evaluation questions and interview? What else might you want to ascertain about her history and symptoms?

2. After reviewing some of the rating scales available for use in your evaluation, please choose one and discuss why you

(continued)

are using this scale, what information it might provide for you, and what you expect the outcome to be.

3. What are your thoughts about her current medications from the PCP and potential for adverse drug effects (ADE) such as tremor, falls, memory, and fatigue?

4. What referrals or interprofessional treatment team members would you make or include in her treatment?

Interprofessional Box

After evaluating a 76-year-old widowed female, your final assessment includes a diagnosis of major depressive disorder, single episode, severe. The patient resides alone in an apartment. She presents as frail, gaunt, and sallow. She indicates that she has experienced a persistent cough and has not been able to get out of her apartment as frequently as she would like due to feeling tired and weak. She indicates that she last went to the grocery store 2 weeks ago. She was brought today to the appointment alone by public transportation.

What referrals would be of benefit to the patient at this time? Consider:

- Primary care provider to rule out medical complications
- Home health—occupational or mental health nurse
- Case management
- Contact adult protective services if no relatives available

Evidence-Based Practice Box

Age-related changes in the older adult can have an impact on various systems of the body that can result in physiological and psychological issues. More than 50% of adverse drug reaction hospitalizations in the older adult are preventable

(continued)

(Lavan & Gallagher, 2016). Thus, complexities related to age-related changes emphasize that providing individualized care rather than protocol-based care is imperative for improved outcomes.

CRITICAL THINKING QUESTIONS

1. When initially meeting a geriatric mental health patient, what preliminary issues might you want to discuss with the patient prior to starting the evaluation?

2. Why would these components be essential to your knowledge prior to assessing their psychiatric symptoms?

REFERENCES

American Psychiatric Association. (2013). *Diagnostic and statistical manual of mental disorders* (5th ed.). https://doi.org/10.1176/appi.books.9780890425596

Folstein, M. F., Folstein, S. E., & McHugh, P. R. (1975, November). "Mini-mental state": A practical method for grading the cognitive state of patients for the clinician. *Journal of Psychiatric Research, 12*(3), 189–198. https://doi.org/10.1016/0022-3956(75)90026-6

Lavan, A. H., & Gallagher, P. (2016). Predicting risk of adverse drug reactions in older adults. *Therapeutic Advances in Drug Safety, 7*(1), 11–22. https://doi.org/10.1177/2042098615615472

Lawton, M. P., & Brody, E. M. (1969). Assessment of older people: Self-maintaining and instrumental activities of daily living. *Gerontologist, 9*(3), 179–186. https://doi.org/10.1093/geront/9.3_Part_1.179

Wong-Baker Faces Foundation. (2016). *Wong-Baker Faces pain rating scale.* https://wongbakerfaces.org/

CHAPTER 3

DEPRESSIVE DISORDERS IN GEROPSYCHIATRY

DEANA GOLDIN

LEARNING OBJECTIVES

After reviewing this chapter, practitioners will be able to:

- define depression
- describe the prevalence, risk factors, and protective factors for older adults with depression
- differentiate between major depression disorder and other mood disorders
- discuss example screening tools to help screen older adults for depression and suicide risk
- describe evidence-based general pharmacological (class) and nonpharmacological treatment options for depression in older adults
- identify barriers and facilitators to promote treatment compliance for older adults with depression

■ INTRODUCTION

Geriatric depression or late-life depression (LLD) is a complex mood disorder that can comprise various etiological pathways and often occurs in the context of medical illness or cognitive decline. Major depressive disorder (MDD) is one of the most commonly diagnosed mental illnesses in older adults and is often underrecognized and undertreated (Maurer et al., 2018; Park et al., 2017). Depressive symptoms are frequently associated with the normal aging process because depression in older adults may be disregarded as frailty, irritability, agitation, or helplessness; therefore, the need to seek medical attention is often overlooked (Okamura et al., 2018). Additionally, age-specific manifestations of geriatric depression are often characterized by hypochondriasis or somatic preoccupations associated with anxiety rather than typical features associated with melancholia or persistent sadness. LLD appearing in adults younger than 60 years of age has a worse prognosis, a more chronic course, a greater relapse rate, and higher levels of medical comorbidity, cognitive impairment, and mortality than earlier onset of depression (MacQueen et al., 2016).

■ PREVALENCE AND ETIOLOGY REVIEW OF SYSTEMS

Due to increasing life expectancy, the burden of depression will increasingly shift toward older age groups; older age groups are disproportionally affected by risk factors such as chronic comorbid health conditions and bereavement (Conde-Sala et al., 2019; World Health Organization, 2016). Older adults are at increased risk for living with chronic medical conditions. Sixty percent of older adults are living with at least one chronic health condition and approximately 42% of older adults are living with at least two chronic conditions (Cheruvu & Chiyaka, 2019). It has been estimated that the population of older adults aged 65 and over will make up more than 20% of U.S. residents by 2030; by 2050, it is estimated that this population will reach 83.7 million (Cheruvu & Chiyaka, 2019).

Depression is not part of the normal aging process; however, depression is prevalent among older adults and requires treatment at any age. Lam et al. (2016) found that depressive disorders were the second-leading cause of disability worldwide. In the United States, the economic cost of MDD in 2010 was estimated to be $210.5 billion (Lam et al., 2016). Depression is associated with high societal and economic burden. Depression can be debilitating when left untreated and has been linked to increased incidence of suicide and decreased physical, cognitive, occupational, and social functioning. Depression is considered a major risk factor for suicide. Individuals aged 65 and older account for 20% of all suicide deaths in the United States, with White males and individuals 85 years and older demonstrating the highest suicide rates (Xiang et al., 2018). It is estimated that more than 2,000,000 Americans suffer from depression (World Health Organization, 2016) with between 10% and 20% of older individuals experiencing a depressive disorder (Avasthi & Grover, 2018). Approximately 52% of patients have their first onset of depression at age 60 or older; for individuals above age 75, the prevalence of depression ranges between 4.6% and 13.5% and increases to 27% in individuals older than age 85 (Burke et al., 2019; Xiang et al., 2018). Fifty percent of older adults with Alzheimer's disease develop a depressive disorder, although it is unclear whether depression is a contributing risk factor or a prodromal symptom of Alzheimer's disease (Balsamo et al., 2018).

◼ RISK FACTORS AND PROTECTIVE FACTORS

Common risk factors associated with depression include past or recent stressful life events, interpersonal difficulties, avoidance or isolation, and anxious response styles (Maurer et al., 2018). Risk factors specific to LLD include (a) being female, (b) being unmarried or widowed, (c) being of low socioeconomic status, (d) having a chronic physical illness, (e) social isolation and loneliness, and (f) a personal or family history of depression (Park et al., 2017).

Older individuals may experience common life stressors; however, some stressors are unique to older individuals. Biological age-related factors increase the likelihood of having medical and physical comorbidities, and depression has a high comorbidity with cognitive decline and other medical and psychiatric diseases. Additional influences for older adults include polypharmacy, altered pharmacokinetics (rate of drug absorption, distribution, metabolism, and excretion), pharmacodynamics (the action or effect of a drug on the body), physical limitations, alterations in cognition, and a variety of late-life events that commonly occur as people age, such as the loss of loved ones. Older adults are vulnerable to physical, verbal, psychological, financial, and sexual abuse, along with abandonment and neglect, which can lead to lasting psychological consequences such as depression and anxiety (Katsounari, 2019). Failure to identify depression in the older adult could have fatal consequences, as inadequate support for depression increases the risk of suicide (Maurer et al., 2018; Okamura et al., 2018; Oluboka et al., 2018; Sachdev et al., 2015).

Protective factors against LLD include engagement in meaningful activities, social support, high sleep quality, physical exercise, healthy diets, effective pain management, and successful treatments of comorbid psychiatric disorders. Access to medical care and other health-related resources are essential to optimize cognitive functions, prevent disease prevention, and support overall physical and mental health trajectories. Depression is less likely to occur if patients maintain a sense of humor, ungrudgingly accept assistance from others, respond kindly to friends and family, show interest in life events, and participate in treatments (Park & Unützer, 2011). Table 3.1 illustrates the changes and symptoms that individuals with depression demonstrate.

TABLE 3.1.
Common Signs and Symptoms of Depression

CHANGE	SYMPTOMS
Change in behavior	Social withdrawal Older adults may not look sad but present looking fearful Less talkative; not willing to engage in conversation Deterioration of self-care Irritability Hypersomnia and/or increased daytime napping Increased alcohol or drug consumption
Change in thought process	Brooding or dwelling on the past Exhibiting self-pity Guilt Feelings of worthlessness Poor concentration
Change from previous optimistic life reference	Helplessness Hopelessness Low self-esteem Lingering sadness or unhappiness

■ DIAGNOSTIC CRITERION FOR MDD AND REVIEW OF SYMPTOMS

Depression is multifactorial in origin and several specific variants for depression can exist in the older adult. Biological, psychological, social factors contribute to geriatric depression; therefore, a thorough biopsychosocial assessment is essential. The U.S. Preventative Task Force recommends screening the general older adult population for depression (Howe, 2020; Maurer et al.,

2018; U.S. Preventative Task Force, 2016). Older adults often misattribute depressive symptoms to old age (Avasthi & Grover, 2018); therefore, older adults often underreport indicators such as adhendonia, loss of interest in activities that used to be pleasurable, uneasiness about the future, poor sleep quality, stubborn and persistent unexplained physical pain, recurrent thoughts of death, and memory and concentration changes (MacQueen et al., 2016; Okamura et al., 2018).

During each clinical encounter, it important to identify any physical symptoms that accompany the patient's condition and consider other medical conditions such as cognitive decline, heart or vascular problems, and metabolic or thyroid issues that may contribute to the patients presenting symptoms (Maurer et al., 2018). Psychomotor retardation is a key feature of geriatric depression that can be assessed by direct behavioral observations of facial expression (flat affect), speech (slow speech with delayed or paused response), eye movement (fixed gaze or poor eye contact), posture (slumped), and bodily movements (slow) (Buyukdura et al., 2011). Depression in the older adult is often connected with cognitive impairment, and dementia is usually associated with apathy and depression (Linnemann & Lang, 2020); therefore, a simple diagnostic approach to distinguish between disorders can be challenging (Burke et al., 2019). Evidence suggests that depressive symptomatology in older adults may be a prodrome for dementia; therefore, cognitive functioning ought to be assessed and monitored regularly (MacQueen et al., 2016; Schneider & Brassen, 2016). Additionally, a drug and alcohol screening should be considered, as drug and alcohol use can attribute to depression and worsen symptoms. Thorough histories from both the patient and collateral sources are of particular importance for this population.

MDD often presents with a combination of depressive symptomology. Criteria for diagnosis include a marked change in previous functioning, depressed mood and/or the loss of interest or pleasure for at least 2 weeks, and at least five of the following symptoms (a) self-reported or observed depressed or low mood; (b) anhedonia or loss of interest or pleasure in activities that were once afforded pleasure; (c) changes in weight or appetite; (d) reported sleep changes; (e) self-reported or observed psychomotor changes; (f) excessive fatigue or somatic complaints; (g) excessive guilt or unworthiness; (h) self-reported or observed cognitive changes such as reduced concentration and attention; and (i) ideas or acts of suicide (American Psychiatric Association, 2013; Lam et al., 2016).

The depressive symptoms of geriatric depression generally have a late onset, occur in individuals aged 60 or older, and may include a variety of symptoms across a continuum (MacQueen et al., 2016). Older adults typically do not present with sadness but instead appear worried, apathetic, and lack motivation (anergia). Amotivation or the inability or unwillingness to participate in health-related activities or social events could be a sign of depression in older adults. An astute clinician will assess older adults for atypical or subtle signs of depressive symptomatology, as older adults may be depressed but not meet the full *DSM-5* criteria of MMD (Avasthi & Grover, 2018).

Due to varying ranges of depressive symptomology depression can be classified as either major and late-life or non-major depression. In the older adult, MDD is considered when a full *DSM-5* criterion is met. Other depressive diagnoses to consider for these individuals include (a) unspecified depressive disorder; (b) clinically significant depressive signs that do not meet full criteria for MDD; (c) "subclinical" depression; and (d) "subsyndromal" or depression without sad or low mood (Avasthi & Grover, 2018; MacQueen et al., 2016). Additional considerations include (a) persistent depressive disorder (also known as dysthymia); (b) bereavement; (c) adjustment-related disorders; (d) mixed anxiety-depressive disorder; (e) depression disorder due to another medical condition; (f) medication or substance-induced depression; (g) vascular depression due to cerebrovascular disease that often precipitates depression in older adults (Avasthi & Grover, 2018; MacQueen et al., 2016).

■ TOOLS FOR DEPRESSION SCREENING

Depressed older adults typically exhibit fewer cognitive-affective symptoms than younger adults. Older adults' depressive symptoms can have wide-ranging presentations; thus, standardized rating scales can be helpful to assess depressive symptoms, independent functioning, cognitive functioning, and quality of life (Lam et al., 2016; Maurer et al., 2018; Okamura et al., 2018). A quick and effective initial screening is the two-question screen. The two-question screen asks, "In the last month, have you been bothered by little interest or pleasure in doing things?" and "In the last month, have you been feeling down, depressed, or hopeless?" An answer of "yes" to either question warrants a more detailed assessment. The PhQ-2 has a sensitivity of 100%, a specificity of 77%, and a positive predictive value of 14% in older adults (Park & Unützer, 2011, p. 6).

Patient Health Questionnaire

The Patient Health Questionnaire-9 (PHQ-9) was the first self-report nine-item questionnaire specific to depression designed for use in primary care (Phelan et al., 2010). The PHQ-9 is available on open access and has been extensively studied as an instrument for screening depression in older adults. The PHQ-9 has nine items that are scored as follows: 0 (not at all), 1 (several days), 2 (more than half the days), or 3 (nearly every day). The nine items are summed, with scores ranging between 0 and 27; a score of 0 indicates that the patient has no depressive symptoms and a score of 27 indicates that the patient is experiencing all symptoms almost daily. A score of lower than 10 has been shown to have an 88% sensitivity and 88% specificity for depression (Phelan et al., 2010). MDD is diagnosed if (a) lower than 5 of the nine symptoms elicited have been present at least more than half the days in the past 2 weeks and (b) if one of these symptoms is either depressed mood or anhedonia (Sachdev et al., 2015). A diagnosis of minor depression is established if (a) two to four symptoms have been present at least more than half the days in the past 2 weeks and (b) if one of the symptoms is either depressed mood or anhedonia (Sachdev et al., 2015).

Suicide Screening

Reported rates of suicide in older adults are higher than in young individuals and psychiatric disorders are present in up to 90% of elderly suicide cases (Sachdev et al., 2015). Suicide risk measures typically have two important goals: to assess both current suicidality and the potential for future suicidal behaviors. Therefore, it is imperative for clinicians to routinely monitor for suicidal ideation and plans in depressed older adults. Suicide is the leading cause of death for depressed individuals with the strongest risk factor being a history of prior suicide attempts (Lam et al., 2016; Yatham et al., 2018). Table 3.2 defines the SAD PERSONS acronym; SAD PERSONS is a mnemonic 10-item scale developed on content validity to assist clinicians in determining suicide risk (Patterson et al., 1983).

As cited in Weber and Estes (2016), The Substance Abuse and Mental Health Services Administration (2018) developed the Five-Step Evaluation and Triage screening tool to identify suicide risk, severity, and protective factors. This tool assesses and documents (a) identifiable risk factors, (b) protective factors, (c) suicide inquiry, including thoughts, plans, and intent, (d) determination of risk or level of intervention, and (e) risk, plan, and follow-up (Potter et al., 2020; Weber & Estes, 2016).

TABLE 3.2.
Suicide Screen: SAD PERSONS

SAD PERSONS SUICIDE CRITERIA	SCORING
S—Male	1 point
A—<19 or >45	1 point
D—Depression of hopelessness	2 points
P—Previous attempt or psychiatric care	1 point
E—Excessive alcohol or drug use	1 point
R—Rational thinking loss	2 points
S—Single, separated, divorced, or widowed	1 point
O—Organized previous suicide attempt	2 points
N—No social support	1 point
S—Sated future intent	2 points
Score 6–8 = emergency psychiatric evaluation; >9 immediate psychiatric hospitalization	

Source: Patterson, W. M., Dohn, H. H., Bird, J., & Patterson, G. A. (1983). Evaluation of suicidal patients: The SAD PERSONS scale. *Psychosomatics*, *24*, 343–345, 348–349. https://doi.org/10.1016/S0033-3182(83)73213-5

■ PERSISTENT DEPRESSIVE DISORDER CRITERIA

Persistent depressive disorder (PDD) is a form of chronic depression that is commonly referred to as dysthymic disorder. Dysthymic disorder was replaced by PDD in the *DSM-5*; the PDD diagnosis consolidates chronic MDD and dysthymic disorder (Devanand, 2014). PDD is considered when an individual has a chronically depressed mood with mild, moderate, or severe depressive symptoms that continue for a minimum of 2 years plus two or more of the following symptoms: (a) poor appetite or overeating, (b) insomnia or hypersomnia, (c) low energy or fatigue, (d) low self-esteem, (e) poor concentration or difficulty making a decision, and (f) feelings of hopelessness (American Psychiatric Association, 2013). While symptom severity may fluctuate, the minimum criterion for PDD is depressed mood for the majority of the day, for most days over a minimum of 2 years (American Psychiatric Association, 2013). PDD is commonly present in older adults without a history of major depression or other comorbid psychiatric disorders. PDD affects men and women equally, and the majority of older adults with PDD have psychosocial stressors such as loss of social support, bereavement, or a cerebrovascular or neurodegenerative etiology (Devanand, 2014).

■ ADJUSTMENT DISORDER WITH DEPRESSED MOOD CRITERIA

An adjustment disorder (AD) with depressed mood describes a maladaptive emotional or behavioral response that primarily manifests as low mood, tearfulness, or feelings of hopelessness in response to an identifiable psychosocial stressor. The psychosocial stressor can be either a single event or recurrent event that occurs within 3 months of the onset of the stressor and results in enormous difficulties in personal functioning and adjustment to the event. Additionally, individuals with an AD respond to the stressor in a way that is considered disproportionate to the stressors' severity. The stressor and the individual's response produce marked personal distress and significant impairment in functioning for a period of less than 6 months that is not related to normal bereavement (American Psychiatric Association, 2013). Risk factors to consider in the older adult population include exposure to actual or threatened death, interpersonal conflict, death of a loved one, financial troubles, or illness of a loved one or oneself. Individuals can be diagnosed with an AD following a death of a loved one if the grief reaction is disproportionate in intensity, quality, or persistence compared to the individual's cultural and societal norms (American Psychiatric Association, 2013). It is important to note that ADs are associated with increased risk of suicide; thus, a suicide assessment is warranted for individuals with ADs.

CASE 3.1

A 69-year-old African American widowed female is brought to her primary care provider by her next-door neighbor who is suffering from osteoarthritis, insomnia, fatigue, and hearing loss. She is seated with a slouched posture and speaks with slow and monotonous speech. She has poor eye contact and mostly looks down at the floor. She is tearful when explaining that she has no energy and no longer attends her weekly card games, book club meetings, and pottery classes because sitting for long periods of time makes her pain worse. She goes on to say that even though she used to enjoy her hobbies and friends, she doesn't care that she doesn't get out of the house much because "it is too much work, anyway." She explains that she does not recall the last time she had a good night of sleep since her husband died 1 year ago. She gets increasingly tearful as she explains that she is nothing more than a burden to her children, feels exhausted, and recalls days where she has too tired to get out of bed. She denies any suicidal ideation or ideas of self-harm but does not feel that her life will ever get any better since. She has tried everything and nothing seems to help with her body pains. She has no past personal or family history of depression or psychiatric illnesses. She does not drink alcohol, smoke, or use illicit drugs. She takes her blood pressure medication daily and uses her hearing aids most days because she sometimes forgets.

1. How would you approach treatment for this patient?

2. What are risk factors to consider for this patient?

3. What are the differential diagnoses to consider for his patient?

4. What are some considerations specific to this patient when formulating her treatment plan?

Interprofessional Box

Patient-centered care includes fostering good communication between patients and patients' team of providers. A long-term, evidence-based, interdisciplinary approach to depression management is best due to the chronic, relapsing, and insidious nature of chronic depression; therefore, interprofessional collaboration between providers fosters ideal patient outcomes. Valuable members of the interprofessional team include primary care clinicians, case managers, psychiatrists, and behavioral specialists. A team-based approach allows for close patient surveillance and enables providers to monitor treatment response, encourage adherence, and offer evidence-based psychotherapies (Van Orden & Conwell, 2016). Age-specific considerations for psychotherapy for the older adult with depression are provided in Exhibit 3.1. The importance of educating patients, families, and caregivers about depression, early signs of relapse, signs of worsening functional impairments, and the importance of routines and regular patterns of activity cannot be overemphasized. Furthermore, it is important to consider the wishes of patients and their families so that clinicians, patients, and families can make informed healthcare decisions that are consistent with patient and family needs, preferences, and values.

Evidence-Based Practice Box

Treating depression in older adults can be challenging in comparison to treating depression in younger populations. Clinicians must aim to recognize and deliver prompt treatment to effectively return a patient to full function. Patient-centered approaches, evidence-based evaluations of the risk-benefit

(continued)

ratios of treatment strategies, and careful monitoring of outcomes are vital to providing optimal treatment that addresses all symptoms and functional impairment, minimizes medication side effects, addresses difficulties to adherence, offers strategies for relapse prevention, and promote patients' dignity, self-respect, quality of life, and overall sense of well-being (Oluboka et al., 2018).

The first-line treatment for geriatric depression consists of nonpharmacological treatments such as environmental and behavioral strategies; however, pharmacotherapy should be considered in more severe cases of depression, especially if psychotherapy is unavailable or ineffective (MacQueen et al., 2016). Treatment plans should ideally be guided by the patient's preferences, previous experiences, core symptoms, safety, and cost-effectiveness. Nonpharmacological evidence-based therapies include cognitive behavioral therapy, mindfulness-based stress reduction, individual supportive counseling, and group therapy approaches. The combination of antidepressant medication, psychosocial interventions, and psychotherapy is optimal for treatment (O'Donnell et al., 2018).

The motto "start low and go slow" is pertinent when considering the use of antidepressant medication. Starting medications in low doses decreases an individual's vulnerability to side effects; the dose should be increased slowly and gradually until a therapeutic dose is reached. Older adults are often underdosed and do not get an adequate response to medications as a result (MacQueen et al., 2016). To be considered an adequate trial, individuals generally take antidepressants for 6 to 12 weeks with close monitoring for side effects and clinical response assessments. Although well tolerated, side effects of antidepressant medications can include gastrointestinal upset, nausea, diarrhea, headache, weight changes, sexual dysfunction, and anxiety. Comorbid treatments and polypharmacy such

(continued)

as drug–drug interactions and age-related pharmacokinetic changes such as decreased absorption and excretion rates for the older adult population should be considered when prescribing medications. Other concerns include potential risk for overdose, sedative effects, cardiac risks, cognitive effects, impact on appetite, anticholinergic effects, and metabolic risks such as hyponatremia (MacQueen et al., 2016). Clinicians must be mindful that medications taken for other health issues can cause or exacerbate depressive symptoms and complicate depression responses to antidepressant medications; thus, a complete review of every medication taken by the individual is warranted. Medication adherence is critical to achieving full, functional recovery; nonadherence can be a major challenge that encumbers the treatment of depression in older adults (Lam et al., 2016).

Selective serotonin reuptake inhibitors (SSRIs) are the most studied and preferred medication for geriatric depression (Howe, 2020). SSRIs are clinically effective for depression and are tolerable and safe for older adults (MacQueen et al., 2016). When initiating an SSRI, it is suggested to begin patients on 50% of the recommended dose and titrate up slowly with frequent monitoring for clinical effectiveness and adverse side effects (Howe, 2020). When prescribing medications, it is important to consider the distinct properties of depressive symptoms in conjunction with safe-prescribing resources in the older adult. The American Geriatrics Society Beers Criteria lists medications that are best to avoid for older adults due to their high-risk profile and serves to improve medication selection, educate clinicians about potential unfavorable drug events, and is intended to improve quality of care and patterns of prescribing of older adults (American Geriatrics Society Beers Criteria Update Expert Panel, 2019, pp. 1–2).

Older adults are at risk for medication-related adverse events; therefore, patient education is essential. For example,

(continued)

fall precautions and driving risks are essential when prescribing medications with sedating properties. Patients should be encouraged to report side effects and ask questions about treatments. Other prescribing considerations include knowledge of how medication side effects can be used to treat depression and improve comorbid conditions. For example, a medication with sedating properties could be helpful to patients with depression and insomnia as well as patients with depression and somatic issues. Antidepressants with pain control properties should be considered when prescribing antidepressants to older adults.

EXHIBIT 3.1

PSYCHOTHERAPY CONSIDERATIONS

Barriers to Psychotherapy

- personal and family perception and attitudes
  - stigma; cultural beliefs; perceptions of being "too old to change"
- transportation challenges
  - patient is no longer driving
  - relying on others to get to appointments; inability for service providers to arrange transport to the clinic
- physical limitations
  - difficulty with sitting for long periods of time and getting in and out of the car
  - ambulatory issues; difficulty with office stairs
- urinary incontinence
  - unable to sit in therapy for long periods without breaks

(continued)

- physical discomfort
  - urge to pace
  - difficulty sitting
- cognitive problems
  - difficulty remembering things
- financial issues
- hearing loss
- lacks family acceptance

Suggestions for Clinical Practice

- adaptability to treatment and structure
- briefer/shorter sessions
- provide written information
- use large font on handouts
- audiotape sessions
- sitting closer to patient
- speak in tones that the patient can hear
- provide take-home materials
- utilize patient's life experiences and unique attributes during sessions
- promote family involvement

REFERENCES

American Geriatrics Society Beers Criteria Update Expert Panel. (2019). American Geriatrics Society 2019 updated AGS Beers Criteria® for potentially inappropriate medication use in older adults. *Journal of the American Geriatrics Society*, *67*(4), 674–694. https://doi.org/10.1111/jgs.15767

American Psychiatric Association. (2013). *Diagnostic and statistical manual of mental disorders* (5th ed.). https://doi.org/10.1176/appi.books.9780890425596

Avasthi, A., & Grover, S. (2018). Clinical practice guidelines for management of depression in elderly. *Indian Journal of Psychiatry*, *60*(Suppl. 3), S341–S362. https://doi .org/10.4103/0019-5545.224474

Balsamo, M., Cataldi, F., Carlucci, L., Padulo, C., & Fairfield, B. (2018). Assessment of late-life depression via self-report measures: A review. *Clinical Interventions in Aging*, *13*, 2021–2044. https://doi.org/10.2147/CIA.S178943

Burke, A. D., Goldfarb, D., Bollam, P., & Khokher, S. (2019). Diagnosing and treating depression in patients with Alzheimer's disease. *Neurology and Therapy*, *8*(2), 325–350. https://doi.org/10.1007/s40120-019-00148-5

Buyukdura, J. S., McClintock, S. M., & Croarkin, P. E. (2011). Psychomotor retardation in depression: Biological underpinnings, measurement, and treatment. *Progress in Neuro-Psychopharmacology & Biological Psychiatry*, *35*(2), 395–409. https://doi.org/10.1016/j.pnpbp.2010.10.019

Cheruvu, V. K., & Chiyaka, E. T. (2019). Prevalence of depressive symptoms among older adults who reported medical cost as a barrier to seeking health care: Findings from a nationally representative sample. *BMC Geriatrics*, *19*(1), 192. https://doi.org/10.1186/s12877-019-1203-2

Conde-Sala, J. L., Garre-Olmo, J., Calvó-Perxas, L., Turró-Garriga, O., & Vilalta-Franch, J. (2019). Course of depressive symptoms and associated factors in people aged 65+ in Europe: A two-year follow-up. *Journal of Affective Disorders*, *245*, 440–450. https://doi.org/10.1016/j .jad.2018.10.358

Devanand, D. P. (2014). Dysthymic disorder in the elderly population. *International Psychogeriatrics*, *26*(1), 39–48. https://doi.org/10.1017/S104161021300166X

Howe, S. (2020, April 20). *Mental health update: Recognizing depression in primary care*. The Clinical Advisor. https:// www.clinicaladvisor.com/home/topics/mood-disorder-information-center/mental-health-update-recognizing-and-treating-depression-in-primary-care/

Katsounari, I. (2019). Older adults' perceptions of psycho-therapy in Cyprus. *Behavioral Sciences (Basel, Switzerland)*, *9*(11), 116. https://doi.org/10.3390/bs9110116

Lam, R. W., McIntosh, D., Wang, J., Enns, M. W., Kolivakis, T., Michalak, E. E., Sareen, J., Song, W. Y., Kennedy, S. H., MacQueen, G. M., Milev, R. V., Parikh, S. V., Ravindran, A. V., & CANMAT Depression Work Group. (2016). Canadian Network for Mood and Anxiety Treatments (CANMAT) 2016 clinical guidelines for the management of adults with major depressive disorder: Section 1. Disease burden and principles of care. *Canadian Journal of Psychiatry*, *61*(9), 510–523. https://doi.org/10.1177/0706743716659416

Linnemann, C., & Lang, U. E. (2020). Pathways connecting late-life depression and dementia. *Frontiers in Pharmacology*, *11*, 279. https://doi.org/10.3389/fphar.2020.00279

MacQueen, G. M., Frey, B. N., Ismail, Z., Jaworska, N., Steiner, M., Lieshout, R. J., Kennedy, S. H., Lam, R. W., Milev, R. V., Parikh, S. V., Ravindran, A. V., & CANMAT Depression Work Group. (2016). Canadian Network for Mood and Anxiety Treatments (CANMAT) 2016 clinical guidelines for the management of adults with Major Depressive Disorder: Section 6. Special populations: Youth, women, and the elderly. *Canadian Journal of Psychiatry*, *61*(9), 588–603. https://doi.org/10.1177/0706743716659276

Maurer, D. M., Raymond, T., & Davis, B. (2018). Depression: Screening and diagnosis. *American Family Physician*, *98*(8), 508–515. https://www.aafp.org/afp/2018/1015/p508.html

O'Donnell, M. L., Metcalf, O., Watson, L., Phelps, A., & Varker, T. (2018). A systematic review of psychological and pharmacological treatments for adjustment disorder in adults. *Journal of Traumatic Stress*, *31*(3), 321–331. https://doi.org/10.1002/jts.22295

Okamura, T., Ura, C., Miyamae, F., Sugiyama, M., Inagaki, H., Ayako, E., Hiroshi, M., Motokawa, K., & Awata, S. (2018). Prevalence of depressed mood and loss of interest among community-dwelling older people: Large-scale questionnaire survey and visiting intervention. *Geriatrics & Gerontology International, 18*(11), 1567–1572. https://doi .org/10.1111/ggi.13526

Oluboka, O. J., Katzman, M. A., Habert, J., McIntosh, D., MacQueen, G. M., Milev, R. V., McIntyre, R. S., & Blier, P. (2018). Functional recovery in major depressive disorder: Providing early optimal treatment for the individual patient. *The International Journal of Neuropsychopharmacology, 21*(2), 128–144. https://doi.org/10.1093/ijnp/pyx081

Park, M., & Unützer, J. (2011). Geriatric depression in primary care. *The Psychiatric Clinics of North America, 34*(2), 469–487. https://doi.org/10.1016/j.psc.2011.02.009

Park, S. C., Lee, H. Y., Lee, D. W., Hahn, S. W., Park, S. H., Kim, Y. J., Choi, J. S., Lee, H. S., Lee, S. I., Na, K. S., Jung, S. W., Shim, S. H., Kim, K. W., Paik, J. W., & Kwon, Y. J. (2017). Screening for depressive disorder in elderly patients with chronic physical diseases using the Patient Health Questionnaire-9. *Psychiatry Investigation, 14*(3), 306–313. https://doi.org/10.4306/pi.2017. 14.3.306

Patterson, W. M., Dohn, H. H., Bird, J., & Patterson, G. A. (1983). Evaluation of suicidal patients: The SAD PERSONS scale. *Psychosomatics, 24*, 343–345, 348–349. https://doi/ org/10.1016/S0033-3182(83)73213-5

Phelan, E., Williams, B., Meeker, K., Bonn, K., Frederick, J., Logerfo, J., & Snowden, M. (2010). A study of the diagnostic accuracy of the PHQ-9 in primary care elderly. *BMC Family Practice, 11*, 63. https://doi.org/10.1186/1471-2296-11-63

Potter, D. R., Stockdale, S., & O'Mallon, M. (2020). A case study approach: Psychopharmacology for atypical antidepressants snap shot. *International Journal of Caring Sciences, 13*(1), 764–769. https://www.internationaljournalofcaringsciences .org/docs/85_potter_original_13_1.pdf

Sachdev, P. S., Mohan, A., Taylor, L., & Jeste, D. V. (2015). *DSM-5* and mental disorders in older individuals: An overview. *Harvard Review of Psychiatry, 23*(5), 320–328. https://doi.org/10.1097/HRP.0000000000000090

Schneider, S., & Brassen, S. (2016). Brooding is related to neural alterations during autobiographical memory retrieval in aging. *Frontiers in Aging Neuroscience, 8,* 219. https://doi.org/10.3389/fnagi.2016.00219

U.S. Preventative Task Force. (2016). *Screening for depression in adults.* https://www. uspreventiveservicestaskforce.org/home/getfilebytoken/BnHj53HwgSBNXMvnyavxfS&dl=1

Van Orden, K. A., & Conwell, Y. (2016). Issues in research on aging and suicide. *Aging & Mental Health, 20*(2), 240–251. https://doi.org/10.1080/13607863.2015.1065791

Weber, M., & Estes, K. (2016). Anxiety and depression. In T. Woo & M. V. Robinson (Eds.), *Pharmacotherapeutics: For advanced practice nurse prescribes.* (4th ed., pp. 897–912). F. A. Davis.

World Health Organization. (2016). *Preventing depression in the WHO European region.* http://www.euro.who.int/en/health-topics/noncommunicable-diseases/mental-health/publications/2016/preventing-depression-in-the-who-european-region-2016

Xiang, X., Danilovich, M. K., Tomasino, K. N., & Jordan, N. (2018). Depression prevalence and treatment among older home health services users in the United States. *Archives of Gerontology and Geriatrics, 75,* 151–157. https://doi.org/10.1016/j.archger.2017.12.005

Yatham, L. N., Kennedy, S. H., Parikh, S. V., Schaffer, A., Bond, D. J., Frey, B. N., Sharma, V., Goldstein, B. I., Rej, S., Beaulieu, S., Alda, M., MacQueen, G., Milev, R. V., Ravindran, A., O'Donovan, C., McIntosh, D., Lam, R. W., Vazquez, G., Kapczinski, F., . . . Berk, M. (2018). Canadian Network for Mood and Anxiety Treatments (CANMAT) and International Society for Bipolar Disorders (ISBD) 2018 guidelines for the management of patients with bipolar disorder. *Bipolar Disorders, 20*(2), 97–170. https://doi.org/10.1111/bdi.12609

CHAPTER 4

BIPOLAR DISORDER IN GEROPSYCHIATRY

HELENE VOSSOS

LEARNING OBJECTIVES

After reviewing this chapter, practitioners will be able to:

- identify diagnostic criteria for bipolar spectrum disorders
- analyze unique differences in bipolar spectrum disorders
- apply assessment tools and differential diagnosis to support bipolar diagnosis
- evaluate risks and comorbidities of geropsychiatric populations with bipolar disorders
- understand treatment options for geropsychiatric populations with bipolar disorder

■ INTRODUCTION

In this chapter, practitioners will be introduced to bipolar spectrum mood disorders, etiology, prevalence, and comorbidities. In addition, this chapter will discuss the differences in bipolar 1, bipolar 2, cyclothymic disorders, and bipolar mixed episodes. A case study will be presented with differential diagnoses and risk factors for comorbidities. Mood disorder assessment tools will be discussed including evidence-based treatment options.

■ PREVALENCE AND ETIOLOGY

Bipolar disorders affect 2.5 million adults in the United States annually, and approximately 6 million Americans have a bipolar spectrum disorder of which 1 million are aged 60 or older (APA, 2013; Sadock, Sadock & Ruiz, 2015; Miller & Lalithkumar, 2013). Lifetime prevalence is 1% for bipolar 1 disorder, as well as 0.5% to 1% for bipolar 2 disorder. Bipolar mood disorders are the sixth-leading cause of disability worldwide for ages 15 to 44 and have increased risks for comorbid substance use disorders, suicide, and other neurological disorders compared with others in this age group. Approximately 1 million older adults with bipolar disorder have a greater burden of medical comorbidity. The average onset is 20 years of age, although 10% to 20% of bipolar spectrum disorder symptomatology present in late adolescent ages. It has been reported that 90% of bipolar spectrum disorder cases occur prior to age 50 and 10% of cases present as late onset, at the age of 50 or older (Carlino, Stinnett, & Kim, 2013).

Epidemiologic studies indicate up to 1% of elderly populations will have a new diagnosis of bipolar 1 or 2 disorder later in life. Up to 10% of older adults, aged 50 or older will have a first manic or hypomanic episode that may not be diagnosed in a timely manner. Misdiagnosis is common in older populations. Overall, most populations will have a previous diagnosis of major depressive disorder and severe symptoms of at least 10 years or longer prior to the correct bipolar spectrum disorder diagnosis. As the world's aging population is growing exponentially, it is predicted that in the next 50 years, populations aged 60 years will triple and the incidence and prevalence of older onset of bipolar spectrum disorder will increase to more than 1 million cases in the United States (Rej, Al Jurdi, & Sajatovic, 2014).

■ DIAGNOSTIC CRITERIA FOR BIPOLAR SPECTRUM DISORDERS AND REVIEW OF SYMPTOMS

The *Diagnostic and Statistical Manual*, Fifth Edition (*DSM-V*) outlines the diagnostic criteria for Bipolar 1 disorder, Bipolar 2 disorder, Cyclothymic disorder, and mixed episodes (American Psychiatric Association, 2013).

Bipolar 1 disorder criteria:

- The disorder is characterized by one or more manic or mixed episodes (the manic episode may have been preceded by and may be followed by hypomanic or major depressive episodes, but these are not required for diagnosis).

- A distinct period of abnormally and persistently elevated, expansive, or irritable mood occurs, and there is increased goal-directed activity or energy lasting longer than or at least 1 week (any duration if hospitalized), which is present most of the day and nearly every day.

- During the mood disturbance and increased energy or activity, there are more than or at least three (or four if irritable mood only) of the following:
  - inflated self-esteem or grandiosity
  - decreased need for sleep
  - pressured speech
  - racing thoughts or flight of ideas
  - distractibility
  - increased activity
  - excess pleasurable or risky activity.

- There is a marked impairment not due to a substance or medical condition.

- In addition, these symptoms:
  - do not meet criteria for a mixed episode
  - cause functional impairment, necessitate hospitalization, or there are psychotic features
  - are not related to substance misuse
  - are not due to a general medical condition
  - are not caused by somatic antidepressant therapy

Bipolar 2 disorder criteria:

- Patient has never had a full manic episode but has experienced at least one hypomanic episode and at least one major depressive episode.

■ There is a distinct period of abnormally and persistently elevated, expansive, or irritable mood and increased goal-directed activity or energy lasting longer than or at least 4 days but fewer than 7 days. It is clearly different from the usual nondepressed mood, as it is present most of the day, nearly every day.

■ During the hypomanic episode, more than or at least three (or four if irritable mood only) of the following occur:

❏ inflated self-esteem or grandiosity

❏ decreased need for sleep

❏ pressured speech

❏ racing thoughts or flight of ideas

❏ distractibility

❏ increased activity

❏ excess pleasurable or risky activity.

■ The episode shows an unequivocal change in functioning, is uncharacteristic of the person, and is observable by others.

■ The episode is not severe enough to cause marked impairment, is not due to substance or medical condition, and there is no psychosis (if present, then this is mania by definition).

■ During the major depressive episode, more than or at least five of the following symptoms are present during the same 2-week period and represent a change from previous functioning. At least one of the symptoms is either depressed mood or loss of interest or pleasure:

❏ depressed mood most of the day, nearly every day

❏ markedly diminished interest or pleasure, nearly every day

❏ significant weight loss when not dieting or weight gain, or decrease or increase in appetite, nearly every day

❏ insomnia or hypersomnia, nearly every day

❏ psychomotor agitation or retardation, nearly every day

❏ fatigue or loss of energy, nearly every day

❏ feelings of worthlessness or excessive or inappropriate guilt (which may be delusional), nearly every day

❏ diminished ability to think or concentrate, or indecisiveness, nearly every day

❏ recurrent thoughts of death (not just fear of dying), recurrent suicidal ideation with or without a specific plan.

■ In addition, these depressive symptoms:

❏ cause functional impairment (e.g., social, occupational)

❏ are not better explained by substance misuse, medication side effects, or other psychiatric or somatic medical conditions

Cyclothymic disorder criteria:

■ The patient experiences a cycling of symptoms for at least 2 years (at least 1 year in children and adolescents) in which there have been numerous periods with hypomanic symptoms *that do not meet full criteria for a hypomanic episode* and numerous periods with depressive symptoms that do not meet criteria for a major depressive episode.

■ The periods of hypomania and depressive symptoms are present more the half the time and the individual has not been without symptoms for more than 2 months at a time.

■ The criteria for a major depressive, manic, or hypomanic episode have never been met.

■ The symptoms aren't better explained by another mental disorder.

❏ Symptoms are not better explained by schizophrenia, schizoaffective disorder or related psychotic/delusional disorder.

■ The symptoms aren't caused by a substance (e.g., medication or drug of abuse) or another medical condition.

■ The symptoms cause clinically significant distress or impairment in social, occupational, or other important areas of functioning.

*Later may meet for bipolar 1 manic phase as it may be superimposed.

What is a mixed episode?

■ Criteria for mixed episode include:

❏ criteria are met both for a manic episode and for a major depressive episode during at least a 1-week period (at the same time)

❑ causes functional impairment, necessitates hospitalization, or there are psychotic features

❑ symptoms are not due to substance misuse, a general medical condition, or somatic antidepressant therapy

CASE 4.1

A 69-year-old male, "Mr. S," presents to the clinic with a 20-year history of major depressive episodes and his chief complaint is, "My neighbor has been looking in my windows."

PAST MENTAL HEALTH HISTORY

Mr. S has had symptoms and treatment of major depressive disorder for the past 20 years if not longer. Symptoms that have waxed and waned for periods of 2 years including periods of him feeling sad with severe depressed mood, insomnia several nights in a row, irritability, poor concentration, either over eating or loss of appetite for several weeks in a row, racing, anxious thoughts, and two previous suicide attempts, at ages 25 and 29.

PAST PSYCHOTROPIC MEDICATION HISTORY

Sertraline (Zoloft), citalopram (Celexa), and fluoxetine (Prozac), venlafaxine (Effexor) were all failures, although he does not remember the effect or why he stopped them. He is now taking bupropion (Wellbutrin) XL 300 mg every morning for the past 2 years.

Psychiatric Hospital History: Mr. S was an inpatient at age 25 for an attempted suicide where he jumped off the roof of his parents' home. The second admission was at age 29; he was drinking alcohol and he was hearing voices and was admitted involuntarily and detoxed off of alcohol.

Social History: Mr. S is divorced; he lives with his girlfriend in a condominium in South Florida. He has been married three previous times and has six children—three from his first wife, two from his second wife, and one from his last wife. There is family discord, and they are not very close, although they do talk on the phone during the holiday season. He has a bachelor's degree in

(continued)

mechanical engineering and has worked as his own boss in construction until age 65; he recently retired after injuring his back at work. He has had legal issues dating back to his teenage years. He identifies as having had difficulty with authority growing up and admits to having had short stints in jail five previous times (none of the charges are felonies). His legal charges were substance use or alcohol use related.

Past Medical/Surgical History: Mr. S has a history of hypertension, dyslipidemia, tobacco use, and takes lisinopril 20 mg every morning and aspirin 81 mg in the morning. At the age of 60, he had a laminectomy, so he takes hydrocodone 10/325 mg two to three times per day for his chronic back pain. For depression, he takes bupropion (Wellbutrin) XL 300 mg every morning and melatonin 5 mg at bedtime for insomnia.

SUBJECTIVE

He endorses his mood as irritable and moody, admits to poor sleep, and reports experiencing paranoid thoughts of his neighbors looking into his condominium windows nightly. He reports symptoms of having a short fuse with temper issues lately, which he feels is related to insomnia (he has only been able to get 3 to 4 hours of restful sleep at night for the past week), which he attributes to paranoid thoughts.

MENTAL STATUS EXAM

Mr. S appears with marginal hygiene, fair to fleeting eye contact, mood reported as anxious, with anxious to constricted affect. He is cooperative, with loud volume of vacillating hyperverbal speech. Thought process is concrete although racing with fixation on paranoid thoughts. Thought content is paranoid; he does not appear to be hallucinating, although upon entry to the room, it sounded like he was talking to someone in the room even though he is in the room alone. He denies suicidal thoughts and does indicate he would fight if someone came into his condominium. Concentration is mildly distracted. Memory remote and recent appears to be appropriate to three-item recall. Insight is limited; judgement is fair to guarded.

Questions:

1. Based upon the limited patient history and current symptoms presented so far, how do you think you might proceed

(continued)

with assessment/evaluation questions and interview? What else might you want to ascertain about her history and symptoms? What treatment could you recommend?

2. After reviewing some of the rating scales available for use in your evaluation, please choose one and discuss why you are using this scale, what information it might provide for you, and what you expect the outcome to be.

3. What are your thoughts about his current medications? Or need for new medications?

4. What referrals or interprofessional treatment team members would you make or include in his treatment?

Differential Diagnoses

Differential diagnoses include major depressive disorder (unipolar depression); schizophrenia or related psychotic (thought) disorders such as schizoaffective disorder, generalized anxiety disorder, panic disorder, substance use disorders; and a general medical condition such as a urinary tract infection or other infection, which in the elderly population is more prevalent. The practitioner will need to complete a full history and physical examination in addition to a mental status examination and a full comprehensive laboratory panel that should include serology such as hepatitis series and rapid plasma regain (RPR) to evaluate for syphilis as this can lay dormant for decades and cause underlying mood, thought, and behavioral changes. Other beneficial testing should include brain imaging and toxicology laboratory analysis (Sadock, Sadock, & Ruiz, 2015).

Key Clinical Assessment Pearls

Diagnosing bipolar 1 versus bipolar 2 is essential as the distinct period of manic symptoms, such as elevated, expansive, or irritable mood, and three or more of the other symptoms listed above would be present most days in a 7-day period to meet for bipolar 1 disorder. For bipolar 2 disorder, the same symptoms would be present although only for 4 days to meet criteria for bipolar 2 disorder. Individuals may still transition to bipolar 1 disorder later in life. To differentiate between bipolar 2 disorder and unipolar major depressive disorder, mood is reported as sad, a depressive mood occurs on more days than not over a 2-week period, and five unipolar symptoms are present. Key clinical assessment would be about sleep disturbances. In bipolar spectrum disorders sleep is lacking, usually for 4 or 7 nights in a row. This insomnia pattern will be reported as less need for sleep, and individuals report about 3 hours of sleep and they do not miss it. Individuals when asked, if they feel rested after 3 hours, they may report they wake up and are ready to go, like their motor is on and ready for the day. They tend to not miss getting 8 hours of restful sleep. For individuals with unipolar major depressive disorder, they consistently report poor sleep, initial insomnia, and difficulty falling asleep or staying asleep. These individuals when asked, will tell the practitioner they miss the sleep and always feel tired in the morning.

When individuals with Bipolar 1 disorder have predominant symptoms, the practitioners will use the chief presenting symptom as specifiers to diagnose the current phase. For instance, the hypomanic phase, manic phase, mixed phase or manic phase with psychotic features. A key caveat is, individuals do not have to have a hypomanic phase to meet criteria for bipolar 1 disorder, just one manic episode.

Risk Factors and Comorbidities for Geropsychiatric Population

New onset of bipolar spectrum disorders in geropsychiatric populations have many risks since this is discovered in 10% of those with mood disorders in populations aged 50 and older. Research shows that bipolar spectrum disorder is a diagnosis of exclusion of organic disease processes secondary to later-age presentation of symptoms. One caveat, late-age presentation of bipolar spectrum disorder does occur as a primary first-time psychiatric diagnosis and it is important to call attention to this fact so that geropsychiatry patients will receive the correct diagnosis and treatment. In addition, bipolar spectrum disorders may present as a mixed mood and thought disorder symptomatology presentation; therefore a good assessment and collaboration with an interprofessional team is very beneficial.

Treatment Options

Psychopharmacology treatment options include valproic acid (Depakote), lithium, lamotrigine (Lamictal) or quetiapine (Seroquel), lurasidone (Latuda), and risperidone (Risperdal) for manic symptoms. Reducing or discontinuing bupropion is an option as this medication may induce manic symptoms, insomnia, and complicate mood symptoms.

Discussion

Approximately 10% of older adults, aged 50 or older, will have a first manic episode. The most prevalently documented presentation is irritability and paranoia. A key clinical caveat is that the first documented manic episode presents in older individuals who have been previously diagnosed with major depressive (unipolar) disorder. Making the accurate diagnosis of bipolar spectrum disorder is impactful and can be life changing. Individuals can have a long sequalae of events if not diagnosed accurately in a timely manner. Older adults who present with bipolar spectrum disorder may present with sub-syndromal symptoms or full manic episode symptoms. Older populations should have a full medical workup, including neuro-imaging, to rule out a medical comorbid condition, as well as a toxicology analysis to rule out a substance use disorder or intoxication. Prompt assessment, evaluation, and treatment are of significant importance secondary to the potential severity of older onset of bipolar spectrum disorder.

Interprofessional Box

After evaluating a 62-year-old male, your final assessment includes a diagnosis of bipolar 1 disorder with new onset of a first manic phase. The patient has had seven nights of less need for sleep or poor sleep, paranoid thinking, irritable mood, mood swings, distractibility, racing thoughts, hyperverbal speech, and previous depressive phases. He indicates he has a history of doing poorly on serotonin reuptake inhibitors (SSRIs) and is taking bupropion (Wellbutrin) a norepinephrine-dopamine reuptake inhibitor (NDRI), which could potentiate manic phases. His medical workup and neuroimaging is negative for a medical etiology. What referrals or collaborations would be of benefit to the patient at this time?

Consider:

- Depression and bipolar alliance organization
- Licensed mental health therapist and/or clinical psychologist
- Primary care provider
- And collaboration in obtaining a release of consent to talk with his girlfriend

Evidence-Based Practice Box

Geriatric populations are treated appropriately according to clinical presentation and severity. Pharmacologic, nonpharmacologic, and complementary alternative health approaches should be considered for a holistic approach as bipolar 1 disorder will present as recurrent phases of depressive, hypomanic, and manic phases throughout someone's life. Bipolar 2 will present as long phases of depressive symptoms, hypomanic symptoms, and cycling may be an incidence. There are limited research studies related to

(continued)

the pharmacologic treatment for geropsychiatric populations exclusively, although most current research studies utilized mixed pools of 18- to 65-year-old populations when reporting on evidence-based approaches. Promoting restful circadian sleep cycles, self-care efficacy, social functioning, and environmental stability is an evidence-based approach to lifestyle change that contributes to remitting symptoms.

Pharmacologic approaches are aimed at treating the depressive, hypomanic or manic, or psychotic phases and symptoms. The most-studied FDA-approved medications in bipolar spectrum disorders are lithium and lamotrigine for depressive or manic symptoms versus lithium as monotherapy or valproate (depakote) as monotherapy; the combination of lithium plus lamotrigine was found to be superior to valproate (depakote) for bipolar manic symptoms. Specifically in geropsychiatric populations with predominantly bipolar depression, FDA-approved fluoxetine (Prozac) and olanzapine (Zyprexa) produced remitting symptoms, although in some cases fluoxetine (Prozac) had to be discontinued secondary to resurgence of hypomania and/or mania symptoms (Malhi, Gessler & Outhred, 2017). In predominantly manic symptoms, FDA-approved antipsychotic medications that were found most beneficial were aripiprazole (Abilify), quetiapine (Seroquel), risperidone (Risperdal), or ziprasidone (Geodon); however, antipsychotic medications in the elderly may contribute to a higher risk for stroke and/or sudden death and are contraindicated in the elderly with dementia neurocognitive impairment (Malhi, Gessler & Outhred, 2017; Stahl, 2017).

First-line pharmacologic medications prescribed for bipolar 1 disorder and bipolar 2 disorder are typically mood-stabilizing anticonvulsant agents, such as valproic acid or valproate sodium or lamotrigine, although they must be prescribed with caution in geriatric populations secondary to hepatic metabolic pathways. Other mood-stabilizing anticonvulsant FDA-approved medications are carbamazepine

(continued)

(Tegretol) or topiramate (Topamax) (Sajatovic, & Chen, 2019). Another non-anticonvulsant medication that is very effective is lithium, or lithobid, although caution must be used in geropsychiatric populations secondary to renal metabolism (Sajatovic, & Chen, 2019).

For patients with predominately bipolar 1 disorder with hypomanic, manic, or rapid cycling symptoms, most antipsychotic medications that are prescribed are aripiprazole (Abilify), quetiapine (Seroquel), risperidone (Risperdal), ziprasidone (Geodon), and newer medications such as lurasidone (Latuda) or cariprazine (Vraylar) although benefits should outweigh the risks and careful selection of patient population is indicated (Gareri, Segura-Garcia, Manfredi, Bruni, et. al., 2014).

For geropsychiatric patients who experience severe depressive or manic (psychotic) symptoms and are not able to tolerate higher doses of psychotropic medications to achieve remission and have refractory symptoms, it was revealed in a subgroup research study that electroconvulsive treatment (ECT) is effective, although follow-up low dose lithium or lamotrigine is recommended for maintenance therapy (Sajatovic, & Chen, 2019). In refractory cases, alternative maintenance medications included aripiprazole (Abilify), quetiapine (Seroquel), risperidone (Risperdal), or ziprasidone (Geodon) based on efficacy in reducing symptoms (Gareri, Segura-Garcia, Manfredi, Bruni, et. al., 2014).

Nonpharmacologic or psychotherapeutic approaches are aimed at treating psychosocial stressors, improving self-awareness and self-esteem, regulating sleep, aiding in adherence to treatment, reducing stigma, all of which allow the patient to process the signs and symptoms of bipolar spectrum disorder. In addition, building relationships and reducing risks for substance use disorders are accomplished with psychotherapeutic approaches. Complementary alternative health approaches such as yoga, sleep hygiene, exercise, and health promotion improve outcomes (Rhoads & Murphy, 2015).

CRITICAL THINKING QUESTIONS

1. When initially meeting a geriatric mental health patient with a history of major depressive disorder and new onset of insomnia and paranoia, what preliminary assessment questions might you want to ask? Why would these questions be essential to your knowledge while developing a treatment plan for their psychiatric symptoms?

2. How will you want to manage the patient? Will geropsychiatric patients require more vigilant monitoring?

REFERENCES

American Psychiatric Association. (2013). *Diagnostic and statistical manual of mental disorder* (5th ed.). https://doi.org/10.1176/appi.books.9780890425596

Carlino, A., Stinnett, J., & Kim, D. (2013). New onset of bipolar disorder in late life. *Psychosomatics, 54*(1), 94–97. https://doi.org/10.1016/j.psm.2012.01.006

Gareri, P., Segura-Garcia, C., Manfredi, V., Bruni, A., Ciambrone, P., Cerminara. G., De Sarro, G., & Da Fazio, P. (2014). Use of atypical antipsychotics in the elderly: A clinical review. *Clinical Intervention Aging, 9*, 1363–1373. https://doi.org/10.2147/CIA.S63942

Malhi, G. S., Gessler, D., & Outhred, T. (2017). The use of lithium for the treatment of bipolar disorder: Recommendations from clinical practice guidelines. *Journal of Affective Disorders, 217*(1), 266–280. https://doi.org/10.1016/j.jad.2017.03.052

Miller, M., & Lalithkumar, S. (2013). *Geriatric psychiatry. Pittsburgh Pocket Psychiatry* (pp. 208–209). Oxford University Press.

Rej, S., Al Jurdi, R., & Sajatovic, M. (2014). Managing late-life bipolar disorder: Current issues and clinical tips. *Psychiatric Times*, *31*. https://www.psychiatrictimes.com/managing -late-life-bipolar-disorder-current-issues-and-clinical-tips

Rhoads, J., & Murphy, P. (2015). Bipolar disorder. In *Clinical consult to psychiatric nursing for advanced practice* (pp. 151–177). Springer Publishing Company.

Sadock, B. J., Sadock, V. A., & Ruiz, P. (2015). *Kaplan & Sadock's synopsis of psychiatry* (11th ed.). Wolters-Kluwer.

Sajatovic, M., & Chen, P. (2019). Geriatric bipolar disorder. *UpToDate*.

Stahl, S. (2017). *Prescriber's guide: Stahl's essential psychopharmacology* (6th ed.). Cambridge University Press.

FURTHER READING

Bressert, S. (2018). Cyclothymic disorder (cyclothymia) symptoms. *PsychCentral*. https://psychcentral.com/ disorders/cyclothymic-disorder-cyclothymia/

Chou, P., Tseng, W., Lin, C., Lan, H., & Chan, C. (2015). Late onset bipolar disorder: A case report and review of the literature. *Journal of Clinical Gerontology and Geriatrics*, *6*(1), 27–29. https://doi.org/10.1016/j.jcgg.2014.05.002

Depression and Bipolar Support Alliance. (n.d.). https:// www.dbsalliance.org/

Ferri, F. F. (2017). *Ferri's clinical Advisor: Five books in one.* Elsevier.

Hirsfeld, R., Williams, J., Robert, L., Spitzer, J., Calabrese, R. Flynn, L., Keck, Pl, Lewis, L., McElroy, S., Post, R., Rapport, D., Russell, J., Sachs, G., & Zajecka, J. (2000). Development and validation of a screening instrument for bipolar spectrum disorder: The mood disorder questionnaire. *American Journal of Psychiatry*, *15*(11), 1873–1875. https:// doi.org/10.1176/appi.ajp.157.11.1873

Lukasiewicz M., Gerard, S., & Besnard, A. (2013). Young Mania Rating Scale: How to interpret the numbers? Determination of a severity threshold and of the minimal clinically significant difference in the EMBLEM cohort. *International Journal Methods of Psychiatry*, *22*(1), 46–58. https://doi.org/10.1002/mpr.1379

National Alliance on Mental Health. (2017). *Bipolar disorder.* https://www.nami.org/Learn-More/Mental-Health -Conditions/Bipolar-Disorder

Young R., Biggs J., Ziegler, V., & Meyer, D. (1978). YMRS: A rating scale for mania: reliability, validity and sensitivity. *British Journal of Psychiatry*, *133*, 429–435. https://doi. org/10.1192/bjp.133.5.429

CHAPTER 5

ANXIETY DISORDERS

LEIGH POWERS
ABIMBOLA FARINDE
MARIE SMITH-EAST

LEARNING OBJECTIVES

After reviewing this chapter, practitioners will be able to:

- define anxiety
- distinguish between generalized anxiety disorder, social phobia, agoraphobia, panic disorder, and obsessive-compulsive disorder
- discuss example tools that can be used to establish an anxiety disorder diagnosis
- assess a geriatric patient for post-traumatic stress disorder using an appropriate clinical rating scale
- recommend general pharmacological (class) and nonpharmacological treatment options for anxiety disorders

■ INTRODUCTION

Just as heart disease has been named the medical "silent killer," anxiety later in life may often also be discounted and considered a quiet psychiatric disorder. Anxiety is often overlooked and dismissed in the geriatric population but can have dire consequences both mentally and physically. Anxiety disorders are postulated to be caused by a combination of factors that include changes in the chemistry of the human brain, environmental stress, and genetic components. There is currently no definitive cause for anxiety disorders but researchers are finding more links about these various factors (Kelly, 2019). Not only are anxiety disorders common in the geriatric population, comorbid medical issues can mimic or overlap anxiety disorders, making diagnosing more complex. In younger patients, anxiety may more often present as the primary complaint. It is more common in older adults to verbalize anxiety complaints through somatic symptoms (Cassidy & Rector, 2008). Later-life anxiety is often found in conjunction with major depressive disorders, and can have foundations in dietary issues as well as drug associations. It is paramount for a practitioner to ensure proper laboratory monitoring to rule out a medical etiology.

There has been a correlation between long-term presence of anxiety in older adults associated with female gender, lower level of educational achievement, being unmarried, and having three or more comorbid chronic conditions (Gum et al., 2009). The most common diagnosed anxiety disorder in the geriatric population is generalized anxiety disorder (GAD). Other anxiety disorders frequently encountered in practice include social phobia, agoraphobia, panic disorder, post-traumatic stress disorder, and obsessive-compulsive disorder. Each disorder will be briefly outlined and discussed below.

■ GENERALIZED ANXIETY DISORDER

Intermittent and in response to certain situations, anxiety is often considered normal and can be expected. However, when anxiety becomes severe, interfering with activities of daily living and functioning, treatment can be warranted. Persons who have generalized anxiety disorder express the sentiment of feeling anxious and nervous all of their lives. According to the *Diagnostic and Statistical Manual of Mental Disorders*, Fifth Edition (*DSM-V*), the diagnostic criteria for GAD include excessive, impeding worry, associated with a variety of physical symptoms that occur more days than not for at least 6 months, is not attributed to the physiological effects of a substance or medical condition, and can not be better explained by another mental disorder (American Psychiatric Association, 2013). The anxiety and the worry can be associated with three out of six symptoms. The individual can find it difficult to control the degree of their worry. In particular, for children only one item is required as part of the diagnostic criteria to meet the diagnosis, and these symptoms can include restlessness or feeling keyed up or on the edge, being easily fatigued, difficulty concentrating or mind going blank, irritability, muscle tension, and sleep disturbance. When it comes to clinical expression it is typically consistent across the life span of most individuals and can lead to substantial distress and disability (Hoge et al., 2012).

Common issues:

- A majority of patients have experienced a previous onset of GAD, now presenting with intensification later in life (Cassidy & Rector, 2008).
- Generalized anxiety disorder as well as panic disorder are often misdiagnosed and instead attributed to physical ailments (Locke et al., 2015).

Tools for differentiating diagnosis:
The core symptoms that can be associated with GAD include fast or irregular heartbeat, headaches, difficulty sleeping, and nausea, vomiting, and diarrhea (Torpy et al., 2011). When it comes to the diagnosis of generalized anxiety disorder, it is important to identify the physical symptoms that can accompany the condition as this may help to rule out other medical conditions such as heart problems or thyroid issues (Torpy et al., 2011). The use of the *DSM-V* aids with establishing the diagnostic features of generalized anxiety disorder and also separates it from nonpathological anxiety (American Psychiatric Association, 2013). The *DSM-V* can serve as a primer too for differentiating generalized anxiety disorder from other conditions. Excessive worry and disruption

is a primary indicator of GAD; the worry that accompanies GAD can be pervasive, pronounced, and distressing to the person (American Psychiatric Association, 2013). Along with the use of *DSM-V*, there are a number of scales to establish the diagnosis of generalized anxiety disorder and its severity. For example, the GAD-7 has been validated as a diagnostic tool and assessment scale (Locke et al., 2015). Some of the screener questions that are included on the GAD-7 include feeling nervous, anxious, or on edge, not being able to stop or control worrying, or worrying too much about different things. Another instrument is the PROM-MIS Emotional Distress-Anxiety-Short Form.

In adults, the Severity Measure for Generalized Anxiety Disorder-Adult assists with the clinical evaluation of generalized anxiety disorder (Locke et al., 2015). The clinical evaluation of the symptoms of generalized anxiety disorder will aid with formal diagnosis.

■ SOCIAL PHOBIA (SOCIAL ANXIETY DISORDER)

Social phobia, also known as social anxiety disorder, is defined as a condition lasting at least 6 months in which people can experience fear in one or more social situations (Anxiety & Depression Association of America, 2020). The disorder was first included in the third edition of the *DSM* in 1980 (Canton et al., 2012). The degree of the anxiety that is experienced is above the proportion of the actual threat that is posed by the situation that is feared. An individual may fear that they will undergo the scrutiny of others if they act in a manner or way that displays their anxiety symptoms, which will be negatively received (American Psychiatric Association, 2013). In children, it is important to note that the anxiety may occur in peer settings and not during adult interaction, or the fear of anxiety can be expressed as crying, tantrums, freezing, or clinging (American Psychiatric Association, 2013).

Common symptoms include:

The hallmark features of social phobia include the marked, intense fear or anxiety of social situations (American Psychiatric Association, 2013). The common symptoms of social phobia can include sweating, blushing, trembling or shaking, fast heartbeat, muscle tension, confusion, or cold clammy hands, to name a few (Tracy, 2020). Clarifying and confirming symptoms, their frequency and their severity can assist in the formal diagnosis of social phobia as well as differentiate from normal anxiety associated with social situations, which does not necessarily constitute a condition that leads to impairment of functioning.

Tools for differentiating diagnosis:

The use of the *DSM-V* is a key indicator for the differentiating social phobia from other conditions. It is viewed as a precursor for agoraphobia so when it comes to diagnosis it should be differentiated in terms of presentation and symptoms from other conditions such as panic disorder, depression, or generalized anxiety disorder (Bernstein, 2018). Besides the use of the *DSM-V* there are instruments that are used in the assessment of adults with social phobia. An example of an instrument is the Liebowitz Social Anxiety Scale (LSAS), the Social Phobia Inventory (SPIN), and the Brief Social Phobia Scale (BSPS). The LSAS is a self-rating scale that has been heavily studied all over for its psychometric qualities (Osório et al., 2012). The SPIN is also a self-rating instrument, which is comparable to the LSAS as it also seeks to evaluate fear and avoidance symptom but it differs in that it also assesses physiological symptoms of depression such as palpitation, blushing, tremor, and transpiration (Osório et al., 2012). Lastly, the BSPS is a hetero-applied instrument that also involves the clinician in identifying and assessing symptoms of social anxiety (Osório et al., 2012). Over the years there has been progress made with validating these instruments so they can be accurately utilized for social phobia.

■ AGORAPHOBIA

Agoraphobia is recognized as a type of anxiety disorder that involves a feeling of fear about being in places or situations from which the individual might find it difficult to escape (Hara et al., 2012). The fear associated with agoraphobia can involve clusters of situations (Hara et al., 2012). According to the *DSM-V*, the diagnostic criteria includes a marked fear or anxiety about two (or more) of the following five: using public transportation, being in open spaces, being in enclosed places, standing in line or being in a crowd, or being outside of the home or alone (American Psychiatric Association, 2013). The behavior of an individual with agoraphobia is to avoid these situations because of thoughts that escape might be difficult or help might not be available in the event of developing panic-like symptoms or other incapacitating or embarrassing symptoms (American Psychiatric Association, 2013; Yasgur, 2018). The fear or avoidance that is exhibited by an individual is typically persistent and lasts for at least 6 months or longer (American Psychiatric Association, 2013; Yasgur, 2018).

Common symptoms include:
With agoraphobia an individual can possess feelings of anxiety that they will have another panic attack. The common symptoms of agoraphobia can include chest pains, dizziness, shortness of breath, dizziness, or diarrhea (Dryden-Edwards, 2020; Medical News Today, 2020). The fear, anxiety, and avoidance can be debilitating to a person and can significantly impair their level of functioning (McCabe et al., 2020).

Tools for differentiating diagnosis:
The diagnosis of agoraphobia is based on signs and symptoms, a detailed interview with a mental health professional, a physical examination to rule out other conditions that can also cause the symptoms of agoraphobia, and the criteria for agoraphobia as defined by the *DSM-V* (Mayo Clinic, 2020). There are currently no diagnostic laboratory tests for agoraphobia and similar phobias so a thorough assessment of the signs and symptoms as well

other subjective and objective information will assist with ruling out other differential diagnoses such as social anxiety disorder, generalized anxiety disorder, or post-traumatic stress disorder (Tidy, 2016).

■ PANIC DISORDER

Panic disorder is considered to be a common and often times debilitating disease in which an individual experiences immediate and unpredictable panic attacks (Friedlander et al., 2004). A person can experience symptoms of overwhelming anxiety and palpitations and there is the constant concern of having another attack. According to the *DSM-V*, a panic disorder is defined as an abrupt surge of intense fear or intense discomfort that reaches a peak within minutes and during the time four or more symptoms can occur: palpitations, sweating, trembling or shaking, sensations of shortness of breath, chest pain or discomfort, nausea or abdominal distress, feeling dizzy, unsteady, light-headed, or faint, chills or heat sensations, paresthesias, derealization, fear of losing control or "going crazy," or fear of dying (American Psychiatric Association, 2013).

The attacks as experienced by an individual have occurred for one month or more with either one or both of the following: persistent concern or worry about additional attacks or their consequences and/or a significant maladaptive change in behavior related to the attacks.

Common symptoms include:
The common symptoms of panic disorder are those associated with a panic attack and these include shortness of breath, dizziness (vertigo), lightheadedness, nausea, feeling lie you are choking, sweating or chills, shaking or trembling, chest pain or tightness, and feeling like you might die to name a few. The experiences can be different from each person and these symptoms can also vary in presentation and severity (Healthline, 2020).

Tools for differentiating diagnosis:

A comprehensive understanding of panic disorders is important, especially for emergency room providers, as patients can present with this condition more frequently than expected. It is reported that about 25% of patients that present to the emergency room with chest pain have a panic anxiety disorder (Memon, 2018). The symptoms of an anxiety attack can mimic the symptoms that are found with life-threatening medical disorders such as myocardial infarction or pulmonary embolus (Memon, 2018). When it comes to making a diagnosis it is important to be mindful of the symptomology of other medical conditions (e.g., angina, myocardial infarction, mitral valve prolapse, asthma, hyperthyroidism, or hypoglycemia.

An example of a diagnostic tool that can be used for panic disorder is the Patient Health Question-Panic Disorder (PHQ-PD), which is a main tool that is currently being utilized due to its good psychometric properties and ease of use and understanding (Munoz-Navarro et al., 2016). The use of the *DSM-V* diagnostic criteria is viewed to be a premier diagnostic criterion for panic disorder along with the performance of a physical examination.

■ POST-TRAUMATIC STRESS DISORDER

Post-traumatic stress disorder (PTSD) is a mental disorder that develops after exposure to a threatening or horrifying event (Bisson, 2015). The reaction that is exhibited to a traumatic event can differ from person to person. Many people are able to demonstrate resiliency and an ability to bounce back following the traumatic event but others may not. PTSD can develop as the result of one traumatic event or from prolonged exposure to trauma (Bisson, 2015). According to the *DSM-V,* the diagnostic criteria for PTSD can apply to adults, adolescents, and children who are older than 6 years of age (American Psychiatric Association, 2013). PTSD is based on exposure to actual or threatened death, serious injury, or sexual violence in one or more situation or event. These include directly experiencing the traumatic event, witnessing the event(s) (in person) as it occurred to others, learning that the traumatic event(s) occurred to a close family member or close friend, and experiencing repeated or extreme exposure to aversive details of the traumatic event(s) (American Psychiatric Association, 2013).

Additionally, there is the presence of one or more intrusion symptoms that can be associated with the traumatic event(s), beginning after the traumatic event(s) occurred. Also, there is a persistent avoidance of stimuli associated with the traumatic event(s), beginning after the traumatic event(s) occurred, as evidenced by avoidance of or efforts to avoid distressing memories, thoughts, or feelings about or closely associated with the traumatic event. Lastly, the avoidance of or efforts to avoid external reminders that can arouse distressing memories, thoughts, or feelings about or closely associated with the traumatic event (American Psychiatric Association, 2013).

Common symptoms include:
The symptoms of PTSD can arise anytime months or even years after the traumatic event.

Tools for differentiating diagnosis: PTSD can be challenging to identify, especially when it arises from an individual's mind. A person can experience memories of the traumatic events that can come back to bother the individual so there can be sleep disturbances, nightmares, or the appearance of flashbacks (WebMD, 2020). There is also avoidance behavior in which an individual avoids people, places, conversations, activities, or even situations that can be associated with the traumatic event (American Psychiatric Association, 2013). The duration of all of these disturbances is to be more than 1 month.

Tools for differentiating diagnosis:
In order to diagnose PTSD, it is important to perform a careful assessment that can include a physical examination, patient interview, and the use of self-report instruments when applicable. The *DSM-V* criteria can be used to identify the diagnostic criteria for PTSD and still remains a gold standard. However, additional assessment instruments can be utilized such as the

Clinician-Administered PTSD Scale for *DSM-5* (CAPS-5). The CAPS-5 is a 30-item structured interview that is used to assess the symptoms of PTSD and make a diagnosis. The PTSD Symptom Scale Interview (PSS-I and PSSI-5) is a 17-item semi-structured interview that is used for the assessment and diagnosis of PTSD (American Psychological Association, 2020). It aligns with the *DSM-V* in its brief format to determine the severity of PTSD symptoms over the past month (American Psychological Association, 2020). Also, the Structured Clinical Interview PTSD Module (SCID PTSD Module) is a semi-structured interview for making major *DSM-5* diagnoses that are administered by a mental health professional taking from 15 minutes to several hours. These example instruments are designed to aid with making a formal diagnosis of PTSD and aid with the determination of possible treatment interventions.

■ OBSESSIVE-COMPULSIVE DISORDER

Obsessive-compulsive disorder (OCD) is thought to be a debilitating neuropsychiatric disorder that has a lifetime prevalence of 2% to 3%. People who are diagnosed with OCD can experience recurrent, intrusive thoughts (obsessions) and/or repetitive, stereotyped behaviors (compulsions) that can last for about 1 hour each day and interfere with functioning (Pittenger et al., 2005). The bothersome thoughts that are associated with OCD can cause significant anxiety, and compulsions are attempts to minimize the intrusive thoughts. According to *DSM-V*, OCD is associated with the presence of obsessions, compulsions, or both that can be time-consuming and cause significant distress or impairment in an individual's functioning (American Psychiatric Association, 2013). The degree of insight, range of symptoms, and severity of these symptoms of OCD can differ depending on the person and thus the therapeutic approach may also differ.

Common symptoms include:
The common signs and symptoms of OCD can include the presence of obsessions, which are uncontrollable thoughts or fears that cause stress, and compulsions, which are rituals or acts that an individual repeats quite frequently. A person may also have trouble controlling intrusive thoughts or behaviors and can spend at least 1 hour per day on these thoughts or behaviors. The symptoms can come and go, reduce over time, or become worse so individuals may find themselves engaging in avoidance behavior (National Institute of Mental Health, 2020).

Tools for differentiating diagnosis:
While the *DSM-V* is regarded as a diagnostic tool for OCD there are additional instruments that are available to make a diagnosis of OCD. The Yale-Brown Obsessive Compulsive Scale (Y-BOCS) is a clinician-rated inventory that is used within the scientific community to shape the diagnosis and research of OCD (Morgieve, 2018). The counterpart for children to the Y-BOC is the Children's Yale Brown Obsessive-Compulsive Scale (CY-BOCS) that includes questions about the presence of various compulsion and obsession items to assess severity (Storch, 2005). Self-report inventories can also be used for OCD assessment but offer disadvantages as they may be completed quickly by the respondent and given to a number of individuals at once (Storch, 2005). It is the culmination of subjective and objective measures that will ultimately lead to a robust diagnosis of OCD.

■ TREATMENT APPROACHES TO ANXIETY DISORDERS

The treatment of anxiety disorder can offer an improved quality of life for many individuals who are diagnosed with the condition.

When it comes to the treatment of different types of anxiety disorders, pharmacological agents (i.e., selective serotonin reuptake inhibitors) are considered to be first-line treatment. However, because selective serotonin reuptake inhibitors (SSRIs) do possess a slower onset of action, benzodiazepines may be given in situations of acute anxiety due to their quicker onset of action (Allgulader et al., 2003). The use of benzodiazepines are not recommended for the management of ongoing anxiety disorders but largely for acute phase anxiety reactions for about 2 to 6 weeks of therapy. When the antidepressant begins to demonstrate its effect, the benzodiazepine is to be gradually tapered off. The use of pharmacology can also be combined with or undertaken as monotherapy with psychotherapy, cognitive/behavioral therapy, support groups, and family therapy. These nonpharmacological interventions can also prove to be instrumental in treating the symptoms of anxiety disorders. The use of pharmacotherapy combined with cognitive or behavioral therapies have been found to be the most effective treatment for certain types of anxiety disorders (Hahn et al., 2008).

While there are few psychotropic medications that are currently approved for use in children, some of antidepressants are used off-label in children. Fluoxetine (Prozac) is approved for use in children to treat depression and SSRIs are considered to be first-line therapies for anxiety disorders (Emslie et al., 2002). The use of pharmacological intervention should not be automatically withheld as they have demonstrated positive outcomes in treating anxiety disorders in geriatric population even though few studies have been conducted in geriatric population. At times it may be viewed as a trial process before the appropriate therapeutic intervention is developed and established for a patient.

CASE 5.1

Mrs. Angela Williams is a 79-year-old Latino American widowed female. She presents to your clinic at the behest of her son. He has brought his mother into the clinic today as she currently is unwilling to drive herself. She fell 1 month ago after slipping
(continued)

on a curb getting into her car after a dinner out with friends. At this time, she finds it difficult to get around in the community without family members' assistance.

Mrs. Williams has been a widow for over 15 years after her husband passed away from complications of congestive heart failure. She has lived alone in a three-bedroom one-story condo 5 miles from her youngest son's residence since her husband's death. She is retired, but worked previously for 25 years as a librarian at the local county library. She now volunteers at the library reading to children once a week. She had been enjoying playing bridge with a women's group weekly; however, approximately 1 month ago she decided to stop attending due to reported "distress about getting around with my eyes, and worry that I might not be able to get home." She has noticed since her eyesight has declined and that she also has been having some difficulty with recall and memory on occasion, which also worries her. She also states she has felt "a bit under the weather," although she was taken to her primary care provider and received a "clean bill of health."

Interprofessional Box

When presenting to a provider, it is not uncommon for a geriatric patient to first see a primary care provider due to primary complaints being of a somatic nature. For the primary care provider, anxious geriatric patients may appear as frail with acute worsening of physical ailments. They may rate their physical health as poor, which can dissuade a primary care provider to consider anxiety in the differential diagnoses.

Mrs. Williams was referred to a psychiatric provider for further evaluation. Over the course of evaluation and treatment, it was noted that the patient continued to report cognitive impairment. Studies have indicated that geriatric patients with cognitive impairment have been noted to

(continued)

have higher levels of anxiety. Evidence suggests the anxious symptoms may increase the patient's risk for worsening decline to dementia (Kassem et al., 2017).

After starting an SSRI, Mrs. Williams was referred to a therapist to treat her anxiety with cognitive behavioral therapy.

■ CONCLUSION

Anxiety disorders are estimated to impact about 40 million adults in the United States who are 18 years and older or 18.1% of the population each year (Folk, 2019). Generalized anxiety disorder is considered to be the most common of the anxiety disorders and it is characterized by an unrealistic or excessive anxiety and/or worry about two or more life circumstances for at least 6 months (Hahn et al., 2008) The hallmark features of generalized anxiety disorder seem to be comparable to many of the other anxiety disorder based on manifestations that consist of insomnia, irritability, trembling, dry mouth, clammy hands, etc. (Hahn et al., 2008). A panic disorder basically consists of an intense fear or impending doom that is intolerable and unbearable; obsessive-compulsive disorder is based on the presence of obsessions (recurrent and persistent thoughts, impulses, images) and compulsions (repetitive behaviors or actions). Also, social phobia (formerly known as social anxiety disorder) is characterized by an individual having a marked and persistent fear of social or performance situations and the exposure inevitablely provokes anxiety that can take the form of a panic attack (Hahn et al., 2008). Lastly, post-traumatic stress disorder typically occurs when an individual is exposed to a traumatic event that is associated with intense fear or horror, and the person persistently experiences the event in the form of nightmares, flashbacks, or intense distress. Depending on the type of anxiety disorder, a treatment plan can be tailored to address the underlying signs and symptoms that may cause significant impairment in functioning.

REFERENCES

Allgulader, C., Bandelow, B., Hollander, E., Montgomery, S. A., Nutt, D. J., Okasha, A., Pollack, M. H., Stein, D. J., Swinson, R. P., & World Council of Anxiety. (2003). WCA recommendations for the long-term treatment of generalized anxiety disorder. *CNS Spectrums, 8*(Suppl 1), 53–61. https://doi.org/10.1017/s1092852900006945

American Psychiatric Association. (2013). *Diagnostic and statistical manual of mental disorders* (5th ed.). https://doi.org/10.1176/appi.books.9780890425596

American Psychological Association. (2020). *PTSD assessment instruments.* https://www.apa.org/ptsd-guideline/assessment/

Anxiety and Depression Association of America. (2020). *Clinical practice review for social anxiety disorder.* https://adaa.org/resources-professionals/clinical-practice-review-social-anxiety

Bernstein, B. (2018). Social phobia differential diagnosis. *Medscape.* https://emedicine.medscape.com/article/290854-differential

Bisson, J. (2015). Post-traumatic stress disorder. *British Medical Journal, 351*, h6161. https://doi.org/10.1136/bmj.h6161

Canton, J., Scott, K., & Glue, P. (2012). Optimal treatment of social phobia. A systematic review and meta analysis. *Neuropsychiatric Disease and Treatment, 8*, 203–215. https://doi.org/10.2147/NDT.S23317

Cassidy, K.-L., & Rector, M. (2008). The silent geriatric giant: Anxiety disorders in late life. *Geriatrics and Aging, 11*(3), 150–156. Retrieved from https://www.researchgate.net/publication/286963396_The_silent_geriatric_giant_Anxiety_disorders_in_late_life

Dryden-Edwards, R. (2020). Agoraphobia. *MedicineNet.* https://www.medicinenet.com/agoraphobia/article.htm#agoraphobia_facts

Emslie, C., Heiligenstein, J. H., Wagner, K. D., Hoog, S. L., Ernest, D. E., Brown, E., Nilsson, M., & Jacobson, J. G.

(2002). Fluoxetine for acute treatment of depression in children and adolescents: A placebo-controlled, randomized clinical trial. *Journal of the American Academy of Child & Adolescent Psychiatry, 41*(10), 1205–1215. https:/doi.org/10.1097/00004583-200210000-00010

Folk, J. (2019). Anxiety effects on society statistics. *Anxiety Centre.* https://www.anxietycentre.com/anxiety-statistics-information.shtml

Friedlander, A., Marder, S., Sung, E., & Child, J. (2004). Panic disorder. *The Journal of the American Dental Association, 135*(6), 771–778.

Gum, A. M., King-Kallimanis, B., & Kohn, R. (2009). Prevalence of mood, anxiety, and substance-abuse disorders for older Americans in the national comorbidity survey-replication. *American Journal of Geriatric Psychiatry, 17*(9), 769–781. https://doi.org/10.1097/JGP.0b013e3181ad4f5a

Hahn, R. K., Albers, L. J., & Reist, C. (2008). *Psychiatry.* Current Clinical Strategies Publishing.

Hara, N., Nishimura, Y., Yokoyama, C., Inoue, K., Nishida, A., Tanii, H., Okada, M., Kaiya, H., & Okazaki, Y. (2012). The development of agoraphobia is associated with the symptoms and location of a patient's first panic attack. *BioPsychoSocial Medicine, 6,* 12. https://doi.org/10.1186/1751-0759-6-12

Healthline. (2020). *Panic disorder.* https://www.healthline.com/health/panic-disorder

Hoge, E., Ivkovic, A., & Fricchione, G. L. (2012). Generalized anxiety disorder: Diagnosis and treatment. *British Medical Journal, 345,* e7500. https://doi.org/10.1136/bmj.e7500

Kassem, A., Ganguli, M., Yaffe, K., Hanlon, J. T., Lopez, O. L., Wilson, J. W., Cauley, J. A., & Osteoporotic Fractures in Men (MrOS) Study Research Group. (2017). Anxiety symptoms and risk of cognitive decline in older community-dwelling men. *International Psychogeriatrics, 29*(7), 1–9. https://doi.org/10.1017/S104161021700045X

Kelly, O. (2019). *What are anxiety disorders?* VeryWellMind. https://www.verywellmind.com/anxiety-disorder-2510539

Locke, A., Kirst, N., & Shultz, C. (2015). Diagnosis and management of generalized anxiety disorder and panic disorder in adults. *American Family Physician, 91*(9), 617–624. www.aafp.org.aap

Mayo Clinic. (2020). *Agoraphobia.* https://www.mayoclinic .org/diseases-conditions/agoraphobia/diagnosis-treatment /drc-20355993

McCabe, R., Stein, M., & Solomon, D. (2020). Agoraphobia in adults: Epidemiology, pathogenesis, clinical manifestations, course, and diagnosis. *UpToDate.* https://www.uptodate .com/contents/agoraphobia-in-adults-epidemiology -pathogenesis-clinical-manifestations-course-and-diagnosis

Medical News Today. (2020). *What you need to know about agoraphobia.* https://www.medicalnewstoday.com/ articles/162169.php

Memon, M. (2018). Panic disorder differential diagnoses. *Medscape.* https://emedicine.medscape.com/article/287913 -differential

Morgieve, M. (2018). A golden standard of evaluate OCD: On the use of the Y-BOCS. *Science Direct.* https://www .sciencedirect.com/topics/nursing-and-health-professions/ yale-brown-obsessive-compulsive-scale

Munoz-Navarro, R., Cano-Vindel, A., Wood, C. M., Ruíz-Rodríguez, P., Medrano, L. A., Limonero, J. T., Tomás-Tomás, P., Gracia-Gracia, I., Dongil-Collado, E., Iruarrizaga, M. I., & PsicAP Research Group. (2016). The PHQ-PD as a screening tool for panic disorder in the primary care setting in Spain. *PLoS One, 11*(8), e0161145. https://doi.org/10.1371/journal.pone.0161145

National Institute of Mental Health. (2020). *Obsessive-compulsive disorder.* https://www.nimh.nih.gov/health/topics/obsessive -compulsive-disorder-ocd/index.shtml

Osório, F., Crippa, J. A., & Loureiro, S. R. (2012). Instruments for the assessment of social anxiety disorder: Validation studies. *World Journal of Psychiatry, 2*(5), 83–85. https:// doi.org/10.5498/wjp.v2.i5.83

Pittenger, C., Kelmendi, B., Bloch, M., Krystal, J. H., & Coric, V. (2005). Clinical treatment of obsessive compulsive disorder. *Psychiatry MMC, 2*(11), 34–43. Retrieved from https://www.ncbi.nlm.nih.gov/pmc/articles/PMC2993523/

Storch, E. (2005). Measuring obsessive-compulsive symptoms: Common tools and techniques. *International OCD Foundation.* https://iocdf.org/expert-opinions/expert-opinion-measuring-oc-symptoms/

Tidy, C. (2016). Agoraphobia. *Patient Platform.* https://patient.info/doctor/agoraphobia-pro

Torpy, J. M., Burke, A. E., & Golub, R. M. (2011). Generalized anxiety disorder. *Journal of American Medical Association, 305*(5), 522. https://doi.org/10.1001/jama.305.5.522

Tracy, N. (2020). Social anxiety disorder (Social Phobia) symptoms. *HealthyPlace.* https://www.healthyplace.com/anxiety-panic/social-anxiety-disorder/social-anxiety-disorder-social-phobia-symptoms

WebMD. (2020). *Symptoms of PTSD.* https://www.webmd.com/mental-health/what-are-symptoms-ptsd

Yasgur, B. (2018). Agoraphobia: An evolving understanding of definitions and treatments. *Psychiatry Advisors.* https://www.psychiatryadvisor.com/home/topics/anxiety/agoraphobia-an-evolving-understanding-of-definitions-and-treatment/

CHAPTER 6

SCHIZOPHRENIA SPECTRUM AND OTHER PSYCHOTIC DISORDERS

MARIE SMITH-EAST

LEARNING OBJECTIVES

After reviewing this chapter, practitioners will be able to:

- recognize characteristics associated with dementia with Lewy bodies as well as early-onset and late-onset schizophrenia
- identify risk factors for schizophrenia
- summarize treatment options for schizophrenia
- initiate a treatment plan that incorporates the nursing process of assessment, planning, implementation, and evaluation for with schizophrenia and other psychotic disorders

■ INTRODUCTION

Schizophrenia is a chronic, costly, and vast (across age groups) mental illness that has a prevalence of less than 1% worldwide with the average potential of life lost as 28.5 years (National Institute of Mental Health [NIMH], 2018a). Individuals with schizophrenia are noted to have increased premature morbidity and mortality compared with the overall population (Saha et al., 2007). Older age is also a risk factor for antipsychotic-induced side effects (Thom et al., 2017) including the risk for falls, QT prolongation, and parkinsonism. A small proportion of older adults experience an onset of schizophrenia after the age of 65, which is rare (Jeste & Maglione, 2013). Hence, proper diagnosis and close monitoring of psychosocial interventions in addition to the effectiveness of medications is warranted.

Psychosis is not an illness (NIMH, 2018b); rather it is a symptom that could be related to numerous disorders. A major disorder that can cause psychosis (or lack of contact with reality) is schizophrenia (recently renamed as schizophrenia spectrum disorders in the *DSM-V*). There are common elements in aging, including a change in thought processes. Some changes occur within normal limits while others may include major clinical features that could warrant concern. Distinguishing whether an older adult has developed late-onset schizophrenia, a medical condition manifesting symptoms as psychosis, or a continuation of underlying schizophrenia symptoms are all integral components to assessment and diagnosis. The purpose of this chapter is to discuss the assessment and treatment of schizophrenia spectrum disorders in geriatric patients.

Review of Symptoms

Several studies have discussed that among older adults with schizophrenia, 20% have a late onset that occurs usually in middle age (after the age of 40; very late onset after 65) while the remaining 80% had schizophrenia since early adolescence/early adulthood (between ages 16 and 30; Folsom et al., 2006; Maglione et al., 2014; Vahia et al., 2010). Symptoms in schizophrenia are discussed as positive or negative symptoms that are characterized by the nature of the symptoms rather than being described as "good" or "bad." Late-onset schizophrenia typically is classified as less severe, with a need for a lower dose of antipsychotic medications and with most late-onset cases occurring in women rather than men, ambiguously attributed to the role of estrogen levels (Castle & Murray, 1993; Howard et al., 1994; Thara & Kamath, 2015).

Positive Symptoms. Characterized as active, exaggerated, ostentatious delusions and hallucinations, suspiciousness, agitated body movements, and emotional dyscontrol (NIMH, 2018b). If the individual has symptoms of schizophrenia for at least a 1-month period but does not have the full 6 months of symptoms for a diagnosis of schizophrenia, the diagnosis that can be given is schizophreniform disorder (American Psychiatric Association, 2013). The diagnosis of schizoaffective disorder includes the presence of symptoms of schizophrenia in addition to symptoms of a mood disorder such as mania (bipolar disorder) or depression (National Institutes of Health, 2018).

Negative Symptoms. Characterized as a reduced expression of emotions (flat or blunted affect), anhedonia, psychomotor retardation, and social withdrawal (NIMH, 2018b).

Disorganized and Cognitive Symptoms. Characterized as extreme confusion, incoherent speech, problems with working memory, and bizarre behavior (NIMH, 2018b).

Assessment of the Geriatric Patient. Various factors must be considered to diagnose late-onset schizophrenia. As Saha et al. (2007) emphasized, late onset (after age 40) has a somewhat better prognosis and requires lower daily dosages of antipsychotics than early-onset illness. Table 6.1 outlines the major differences attributed to dementia with Lewy bodies, early-onset schizophrenia, and late-onset schizophrenia.

TABLE 6.1
Defining Characteristics of Dementia With Lewy Bodies, Early-Onset Schizophrenia, and Late-Onset Schizophrenia

CHARAC-TERISTIC	DEMENTIA WITH LEWY BODIES	EARLY-ON-SET SCHIZO-PHRENIA (BEFORE AGE 40)	LATE-ONSET SCHIZO-PHRENIA (AFTER AGE 40)
Common type of hallucinations	Visual	Auditory	Auditory
Common type of delusions	Not bizarre	Bizarre	Bizarre
Cognitive thinking/alertness	Fluctuating	Consistent	Consistent
History of psychosis	Rare	Common	Family history
Length of time for maintenance on antipsychotic medications	Brief	Long term	Long term
Daily neuroleptic dose	High	Lower	Lowest

Source: Data from Mayo Clinic. (2017). *Dementia with Lewy bodies.* https://www.mayoclinic.org/diseases-conditions/lewy-body-dementia/diagnosis-treatment/drc-20352030; Wetherell, J. L., & Jeste, D. V. (2004). Older adults with schizophrenia. *Elder Care, 3,* 8–11.

Terms and Definitions. Since the implementation of the *DSM-V*, the term for schizophrenia is now referred to as schizophrenia spectrum disorder with the various specifiers that were previously present, such as paranoid, catatonic, undifferentiated, residual, and disorganized types, now excluded as it was deemed that such subtypes were not additionally helpful in providing individualized treatment (American Psychiatric Association, 2013). To meet the diagnosis of schizophrenia according to the *DSM-V*, the individual must have experienced at least two of the following symptoms: hallucinations, delusions, disorganized speech, disorganized or catatonic behavior, and negative symptoms. At least one of the symptoms must be the presence of delusions, hallucinations, or disorganized speech. Disturbances (including social or occupational detestation) must be continuous over at least 6 months during which the individual must have experienced active symptoms for at least 1 month. Symptoms must not be attributed to any other medical condition.

Differential Diagnoses. The following list of differential diagnoses is not meant to be exhaustive; however, the purpose is to illuminate that there are various conditions that can exist alternatively to a schizophrenia late-onset diagnosis. For example, delirium, dementia with Lewy bodies, drug-induced psychotic disorder, major depressive disorder with psychotic features, bipolar disorder with psychotic features, or psychotic disorder due to a medical condition could be diagnosed based on the onset, comorbidities, medications, metabolic issues, severity, and the history of the patient's illness.

Sensory Deficits. As individuals age, there can be sensory changes that affect taste, smell, touch, hearing, and vision. According to the National Center for Health Statistics (2010), vision and hearing impairments double with increased age. Such sensory changes can affect the way in which the individual interacts with their environment daily. Reassessment of the patient's environment and interactions with their environment are necessary to rule out other alternative or contributing factors to the patient's present condition.

Risk Factors

Related to the pathophysiology of schizophrenia, individuals with an increased size in their third and lateral ventricles and smaller medial temporal lobe are at a higher risk for schizophrenia

(DiPiro et al., 2014). Other risk factors include having a family history of schizophrenia, interactions between genetics and the environment such as exposure to viruses affecting the regulation of the immune system (increased immune system activation), pregnancy and birth complications, and psychosocial factors including early mind-altering drug use during teen years/young adulthood (Mayo Clinic, 2017; NIMH, 2018b).

The Role of the Family in Assessment. Family members or caregivers often offer additional insight into the patient's course of treatment and symptoms. While information regarding previous hospitalizations, adherence, response to certain medications, and suspected onset are beneficial, family members or caregivers may not have a full understanding of possible psychiatric diagnoses of which education may be warranted. A balance of listening, understanding the family member or caregiver(s) perception of the illness, and knowledge of previous treatment(s) are key components to devising/recommending an individualized treatment plan that is more likely to be successful.

Cultural and Religious Factors. An often overlooked aspect of treatment related to schizophrenia involves the assessment of the role of cultural and religious factors affecting the individual's life. Grover et al. (2014) explained that religion can not only be an aspect of treatment that instills hope but also can influence adherence and treatment outcomes, particularly as religious delusions tend to held with more conviction than others. Thus, assessing the patient's beliefs regarding the use of medications, particularly among their culture and in regards to religion, could provide additional insight into the approach to treatment. Ensuring that the patient's spiritual needs are met (whether through access to a pastor/priest/religious advisor in person or by phone or transportation to church activities) is a component that could contribute to positive coping outcomes.

Pathophysiology

The pathophysiology of schizophrenia has been attributed to an excess or deficiency related to neurotransmission abnormalities such as abnormal activity at dopamine receptor sites (a hyperactive dopaminergic system, particularly at D2; Patel et al., 2014). Negative symptoms and extrapyramidal (motor) symptoms are attributed to a low level of dopamine and positive symptoms in the presence of excess dopamine (Lavretsky, 2008). Other neurotransmitters involved in the theories related to the symptoms of schizophrenia include glutamate and serotonin, where medications that blocked serotonin receptors were found to alleviate negative symptoms of schizophrenia and in the presence of drugs such as phencyclidine and ketamine (N-methyl-D-aspartate or NMDA/glutamate antagonists), symptoms of schizophrenia are induced (Patel et al., 2014).

Treatment

A unique component that advanced practice nurses can offer to patients receiving treatment for psychosis is the holistic approach to care. Table 6.2 outlines a nursing process checklist that essentially summarizes how to approach treatment. Guidelines for the use of antipsychotic medications are judicious (CMS, 2013) and often refer to symptoms that are distressing or pose a risk of safety to others. Most organizational policies and standard procedures require the use of nonpharmacological interventions such as considerations of the environment or behavioral strategies (Wetherell & Jeste, 2004). If medication is warranted, the lowest effective dose must be used. Atypical antipsychotic medications or Haldol in the short term are medications that may be used to treat psychosis; however, the selection of medication should be based on the individual properties of the medication, adjusted accordingly for geriatrics, and the context of the patient's symptoms (Thom et al., 2017).

TABLE 6.2
Utilizing the Nursing Process Checklist (Assessment, Planning, Implementation, Evaluation)

QUESTION	YES	NO
Assessed physical and psychosocial needs?		
Derived a plan of care suitable to meet the individual's needs?		
Implemented treatment considering standard procedures and organizational policies?		
Determined physical and social outcomes (such as did the patient return to baseline)?		
If you answered no to any of the above questions, go back through the checklist and complete each task.		

CASE 6.1   **THE MAN WITH PSYCHOSIS WHO CONTINUES TO HAVE SYMPTOMS**

A 65-year-old Caucasian male presents with confusion and psychosis (specifically, auditory and visual hallucinations with paranoia) of which his caregiver reports he feels he has had no improvement in symptoms on antipsychotic medication trials of before in the past.

1. How would you approach treatment for this patient?

2. What type of assessments would you complete?

3. What labs would you order and medications (if warranted)?

Interprofessional Box

After evaluating a 65-year-old Caucasian male and conferring with the patient's neurologist, the patient's final assessment includes a diagnosis of dementia with Lewy bodies. His wife, who is his primary caregiver, and his adult children are asking what will this all mean for their family. What other referrals or collaborations would be beneficial to the patient at this time? Consider:

- Referral for resources through local dementia and caregiving associations such as the Alzheimer's Association
- Support groups for caregivers
- Referral for case management/social services
- Licensed mental health therapist and/or clinical psychologist
- Primary care provider

Evidence-Based Practice Box

Treatment for older adults with schizophrenia involves psychosocial interventions that build on cognitive behavioral social skills in addition to antipsychotic medications that are typically administered in lower doses and from the atypical antipsychotic medication category for fewer parkinsonian side effects (Bartels et al., 2002; Jeste & Maglione, 2013). Treatment is often hopeful in the long term as it is not uncommon for sustained remission to occur in older adults with schizophrenia particularly if they have had appropriate treatment and psychosocial support over the course of the illness (Jeste & Maglione, 2013). Close attention to monitoring for adverse effects of medications in addition to utilizing lower doses that are also cost-effective is imperative. Furthermore, alternatives to treatment that would result in less long-term hospitalization involve community support programs that are integrative for family members and provide social/vocational skills training for the older adult patient, leading to beneficial long-term outcomes.

REFERENCES

American Psychiatric Association. (2013). *Diagnostic and statistical manual of mental disorder* (5th ed.). https://doi.org/10.1176/appi.books.9780890425596

Bartels, S. J., Dums, A. R., Oxman, T. E., Schneider, L. S., Areán, P. A., Alexopoulos, G. S., & Jeste, D. V. (2002). Evidence-based practices in geriatric mental health care. *Psychiatric Services*, 53(11), 1419–1431. https://doi.org/10.1176/appi.ps.53.11.1419

Castle, D. J., & Murray, R. M. (1993). The epidemiology of late-onset schizophrenia. *Schizophrenia Bulletin*, 19(4), 691–700. https://doi.org/10.1093/schbul/19.4.691

Centers for Medicare & Medicaid Services (CMS) (2013). Dementia care in nursing homes. Retrieved from https://www.cms.gov/Medicare/Provider-Enrollment-and-Certification/SurveyCertificationGenInfo/Downloads/SC-Letter-13-35-Advanced-Copy.pdf

DiPiro, J. T., Talbert, R. L., Yee, G. C., Matzke, G. R., Wells, B. G., & Posey, L. M. (Eds.). (2014). *Pharmacotherapy: A pathophysiologic approach (Vol. 6)*. McGraw-Hill Education.

Folsom, D. P., Lebowitz, B. D., Lindamer, L. A., Palmer, B. W., Patterson, T. L., & Jeste, D. V. (2006). Schizophrenia in late life: Emerging issues. *Dialogues in Clinical Neuroscience*, 8(1), 45–52.

Grover, S., Davuluri, T., & Chakrabarti, S. (2014). Religion, spirituality, and schizophrenia: A review. *Indian journal of psychological medicine, 36*(2), 119–124.

Howard, R., Almeida, O., & Levy, R. (1994). Phenomenology, demography and diagnosis in late paraphrenia. *Psychological Medicine*, 24(2), 397–410. https://doi.org/10.1017/S0033291700027379

Jeste, D. V., & Maglione, J. E. (2013). Treating older adults with schizophrenia: Challenges and opportunities. *Schizophrenia Bulletin*, 39(5), 966–968. https://doi.org/10.1093/schbul/sbt043

Lavretsky, H. (2008). History of schizophrenia as a psychiatric disorder. In K. T. Mueser & D. V. Jeste (Eds.), *Clinical Handbook of Schizophrenia* (p. 1). The Guilford Press.

Maglione, J. E., Thomas, S. E., & Jeste, D. V. (2014). Late-onset schizophrenia: Do recent studies support categorizing LOS as a subtype of schizophrenia? *Current Opinion in Psychiatry*, *27*(3), 173. https://doi.org/10.1097/YCO.0000000000000049

Mayo Clinic. (2017). *Schizophrenia*. https://www.mayoclinic.org/diseases-conditions/schizophrenia/symptoms-causes/syc-20354443

National Center for Health Statistics. (2010). *Vision, hearing, balance, and sensory impairment in Americans aged 70 and over: United States, 1999-2006*. https://www.cdc.gov/nchs/products/databriefs/db31.htm

National Institute of Mental Health. (2018a). *What is psychosis?* https://www.nimh.nih.gov/health/topics/schizophrenia/raise/what-is-psychosis.shtml

National Institute of Mental Health. (2018b). *Schizophrenia*. https://www.nimh.nih.gov/health/statistics/schizophrenia.shtml

National Institutes of Health. (2018). *Schizoaffective disorder*. https://ghr.nlm.nih.gov/condition/schizoaffective-disorder

Patel, K. R., Cherian, J., Gohil, K., & Atkinson, D. (2014). Schizophrenia: Overview and treatment options. *Pharmacy and Therapeutics*, *39*(9), 638.

Saha, S., Chant, D., & McGrath, J. (2007). A systematic review of mortality in schizophrenia: Is the differential mortality gap worsening over time? *Archives of General Psychiatry*, *64*(10), 1123–1131. https://doi.org/10.1001/archpsyc.64.10.1123

Thara, R., & Kamath, S. (2015). Women and schizophrenia. *Indian Journal of Psychiatry*, *57*(Suppl. 2), S246. http://www.indianjpsychiatry.org

Thom, R. P., Mock, C. K., & Teslyar, P. (2017). Delirium in hospitalized patients: Risks and benefits of antipsychotics. *Cleveland Clinic Journal of Medicine*, *84*(8), 616–622. https://doi.org/10.3949/ccjm.84a.16077

Vahia, I. V., Palmer, B. W., Depp, C., Fellows, I., Golshan, S., Kraemer, H. C., & Jeste, D. V. (2010). Is late-onset schizophrenia a subtype of schizophrenia? *Acta Psychiatrica Scandinavica, 122*(5), 414–426. https://doi.org/10.1111/j.1600-0447.2010.01552.x

Wetherell, J. L., & Jeste, D. V. (2004). Older adults with schizophrenia. *Elder Care, 3*, 8–11.

CHAPTER 7

SLEEP–WAKE DISORDERS

LEIGH POWERS

LEARNING OBJECTIVES

After reviewing this chapter, practitioners will be able to:

- identify the basic physiological states of sleep
- understand the importance of an electroencephalogram in sleep disorders
- define insomnia disorder and the associated diagnostic criteria
- identify differences between insomnia disorders and obstructive sleep apneas
- identify how histamine and melatonin receptors work in sleep disorders
- evaluate the use of common sleep aids in geriatric mental health patients

■ INTRODUCTION

In this chapter, common sleep–wake disorders encountered in the geriatric population will be reviewed. Practitioners will initially learn about normal, basic sleep architecture before being introduced to some of the commonly encountered abnormal sleep issues constituting sleep–wake disorders. This chapter will review tools that can be used to assess sleep and appropriate interprofessional collaboration and referrals.

■ SLEEP–WAKE DISORDERS

Sleep disruption is a common occurrence for adults, with insomnia symptoms reported by as many as 33% to 50% of adults (Buysse et al., 2017). In the geriatric population, sleep dysfunction is frequently identified as a distressing symptom, often one of the most common complaints by elderly patients to their primary care providers. Other complaints associated with poor sleep include daytime fatigue, poor focus and concentration, low energy, depressed mood, and problems with interpersonal relationships.

Insomnia presents itself equally in both men and women; however, evidence indicates a higher incidence in men over the age of 85 (Foley et al., 1999). Other risk factors include comorbid medical issues such as nocturia, hypertension, depression, as well as widow status, lower income, and lower education. In geriatric patients, insomnia itself can increase the risk for accidents and falls, cognitive decline, diabetes, and higher rates of mortality (Kamel & Gammack, 2006).

What is commonly referred to as "sleep" actually consists of progressive repetitive stages termed nonrapid eye movement (non-REM) stages and rapid eye movement (REM) stages (Figure 7.1). In normal sleep, the brain cycles through different levels of activity. There are several stages included in non-REM sleep. During the first stage, which lasts only minutes, the brain is in light sleep and eye movements start to decrease. In the second stage, sleep remains light, but heart rate and breathing begin to slow and the muscles start to relax. As body temperature drops, eye movements cease. Brain activity tends to continue to slow, but noticeable brief eruptions occur. It should be noted that the majority of sleep time is spent in stage 2 non-REM sleep during the sleep cycle repetitions than in any other. In stage three of non-REM sleep, the restorative sleep occurs. These stages occur more frequently in the beginning of the night. Approximately 90 minutes after initiation of sleep, sleep enters REM. Eye movement occurs and brain activity increases to levels near when alert and awake. In addition, breathing rate increases along with more

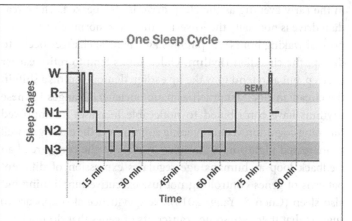

FIGURE 7.1 Stages of sleep. The stages of sleep consist of non-REM 1, non-REM 2, non-REM 3, and REM sleep. REM, rapid eye movement.

SOURCE: WebMD. (2020, January). *An overview of insomnia.* https://www.webmd.com/sleep-disorders/insomnia-causes#1

muscle rigidity and elevated blood pressure and pulse. Although some dreams occur in non-REM, patients primarily will have dream states during REM. This stage is most like being awake, but the body is considered paralyzed and limited in movement. With aging, the stage that tends to shorten most is the REM stage (National Institute of Neurological Disorders and Stroke, 2019). In older adults, it has been estimated that stage 1 accounts for approximately 18% of sleep time, stage 2 for 48% , stage 3 for 16%, and REM for 18% (Wennberg et al., 2013).

Normally, the circadian rhythm creates a natural diurnal sleep–wake cycle in conjunction with the sleep–wake homeostatic drive. The circadian rhythm control center, the suprachiasmatic nucleus (SCN), can be found in the hypothalamus. The SCN regulates many bodily functions that have a diurnal cycle including temperature, heart rate, and the release of hormones related to sleep such as melatonin. The circadian drive is normally highest in the early evening as the sleep drive is also peaked. The circadian drive is normally the lowest in the early morning just before normal waking hours. As patients age, natural changes occur to disrupt the circadian rhythm. Older adults tend to retire earlier to sleep, but also tend to wake up earlier, demonstrating a shift in the circadian clock (suprachiasmatic nucleus). Changes in these rhythms have contributed to noticeable increases in improved morning cognition versus evening cognition in the elderly as well as increased nighttime agitation. Changes in the core circadian feedback loop as humans age regulates expression of different patterns of genes controlling not just executive functioning but also sleep (Chen & Yang, 2015). New evidence also appears to suggest that there are some transcripts of genes that do not activate until older age, possibly attempting to act as a compensatory mechanism for the loss of the normal circadian rhythm processes during aging (Chen & Yang, 2015).

Older adults often have the following complaints:

- increased awakenings throughout the night
- needing to sleep earlier in the evening hours
- reduction in non-REM sleep stages
- early morning waking
- chronic fatigue

In the geriatric population, patients commonly complain of more difficulty with initiating sleep and middle insomnia rather than late insomnia. It is a normal part of aging to see a reduction in sleep duration. Criteria for Insomnia includes the following:

- trouble initiating or maintaining sleep
- daytime impairment in functioning due to missed or unrestful sleep
- daytime impairment may include fatigue, mood disturbance, daytime sleepiness, amotivation, anergia, increased errors or accidents when driving or working, tension headaches, attention, concentration and memory impairment, social or work dysfunction (Sateia et al., 2017)

Common disorders and conditions in the geriatric population that may affect their sleep include other than sleep disorders:

- restless leg syndrome
- periodic limb movement disorders
- cardiovascular disorders—heart failure, nocturnal angina
- pulmonary disorders—allergic rhinitis, asthma
- gastrointestinal disorders—gastroesophageal reflux disease, diarrhea, constipation, IBS
- urinary—urinary retention, nocturia, incontinence
- psychiatric—depressive disorders, bipolar disorders, psychotic disorders, dementia, delirium
- narcolepsy
- behavioral issues—daytime napping, sedentary, smoking, heavy meals
- environmental issues—watching TV in bed, noise, excessive light, bedding
- medications—stimulants (caffeine, nicotine, amphetamines, ephedrine, decongestants)
- antidepressants—Wellbutrin, SSRIs, Effexor
- antihistamines
- alcohol
- steroids

(Kamel & Gammack, 2006)

Other Commonly Seen Sleep Disorders

Circadian Rhythm Sleep Disorder

- Sleep disorders that occur when the body's sleep–wake rhythms are not in sync with light-darkness cycles.
- Continuous or occasional disruption of sleep patterns often associated with complaints of insomnia periodically and excessive sleepiness at other times.

■   Shift work sleep disorder (work schedule conflict with natural circadian rhythms) and narcolepsy (excessive daytime
sleepiness and falling asleep during daytime despite appropriate night sleeping) both fall under these disorders.

Obstructive Sleep Apnea (OSA)

■   OSA disrupts sleep due to the obstruction of the airway,
causing sudden nighttime awakenings.

■   Other symptoms of OSA include daytime fatigue, snoring,
headaches, difficulty waking in the morning.

(Mayo Clinic, 2019).

The goal of the treatment of sleep disorders should be improved
quality and quantity of sleep. Table 7.1 is a list of appropriate
questions for taking a sleep history. Treatment should initially
focus on nonpharmacological interventions. Pharmacological

TABLE 7.1
Questions for Sleep History

1. How would you describe the quality of your sleep?
2. How long do you sleep on average?
3. How many times per night do you wake up? Are there any reasons that you wake up—noise, bathroom, light?
4. How long does it take to fall asleep?
5. Do you wake feeling refreshed?
6. What medications do you take prior to going to bed?
7. How often do you drink alcohol or use any other substances such as nicotine?
8. Any past treatment or medications that have been helpful?
9. What are your pre-bedtime activities?
10. What is your bedroom like—the lighting, TV?
11. Is there a difference in feeling sleepy versus fatigued in the daytime? Are you napping? Do you have problems at work focusing or staying on task? What typical exercise do you do during the day?

treatments may be initiated, but patients should still be encouraged to use nonpharmacological treatment options in conjunction with medications. Table 7.2 is an outline of evidence-based treatments for sleep disorders.

TABLE 7.2
Evidence-Based Treatments for Sleep Disorders (Nonpharmacological and Pharmacological)

SLEEP HYGIENE
The goal of a discussion of sleep hygiene is to limit extraneous factors in sleep disturbance and improve regular sleep routine.
1. Decrease light in the room.
2. Limit electronics 1 hour prior to sleep onset.
3. Keep room cool.
4. Limit activities in the bed to sleeping and sexual activity.
5. No alcohol or nicotine prior to bedtime.
6. Decrease caffeine intake throughout the day.
7. Increase daytime physical activity.
8. Increase light during daytime hours.
9. No napping during daytime.
COGNITIVE BEHAVIORAL THERAPY–INSOMNIA (CBT-I)
The goal of CBT-I is to improve sleep using a structured behavioral program to identify beliefs and behaviors that cause sleep problems or worsen sleep. CBT-I often includes the use of a sleep diary to track behaviors and cognitions surrounding sleep habits.
1. Behavioral control—limiting stimuli
2. Sleep restriction—reduce time in bed when not sleeping
3. Sleep hygiene—as above
4. Environment—review environmental factors to sleep problems

(continued)

TABLE 7.2
Evidence-Based Treatments for Sleep Disorders
(Nonpharmacological and Pharmacological) (*continued*)

5. Relaxation training
6. Biofeedback—gaining insight to feedback from the body such as heart rate and muscle tension
Mayo Clinic (2019)
Antidepressants
■ Trazodone—often used off-label in low doses for its hypnotic properties. Common adverse side effects include gastrointestinal problems, headache, agitation, hypotension, tachycardia, and dry mouth. Caution should be used in the elderly. However, of the older tricyclic antidepressants, trazodone appears to have fewer cardiovascular risks (Stahl, 2017). Doses range from 50 to 300 mg typically for sleep.
■ Remeron—often used with depressed patients with insomnia. Remeron is classified as a serotonin-norepinephrine reuptake inhibitor (SNRI). Start at low doses and monitor for over sedation, tachycardia, and weight gain (Stahl, 2017). Doses range from 7.5 to 45 mg.
BENZODIAZEPINES
■ Benzodiazepines are not advised for long-term use for insomnia with geriatric patients. They are listed on the BEERS list and are advised to not prescribe due to the risk of over-sedation, falls, and cognitive impairment (American Geriatrics Society Beers Criteria Update Expert Panel, 2019). Examples of benzodiazepines include Valium (diazepam), Xanax (alprazolam), Klonopin (clonazepam), Ativan (lorazepam), and Librium (chlordiazepoxide).
NONBENZODIAZEPINE SLEEP AIDS
■ Ramelteon (Remeron)
■ Zolpidem (Ambien, Ambien CR)
■ Eszopiclone (Lunesta)
■ Zaleplon (Sonata)

(continued)

TABLE 7.2
Evidence-Based Treatments for Sleep Disorders (Nonpharmacological and Pharmacological) (*continued*)

HISTAMINE RECEPTOR BLOCKERS
Antihistamines, such as hydroxyzine and diphenhydramine, have been used for their sedative effects for sleep. However, histamine blockers also include high risks of cognitive impairment, risk of falls, daytime drowsiness, and anticholinergic effects that should typically be avoided in the elderly.

MELATONIN
There are not many large-scale studies related to the use of melatonin in the elderly. There have been several short-term small clinical trials demonstrating efficacy for insomnia in the elderly. However, the medication is an over-the-counter sleep aid and does not include FDA regulation. Therefore, dosing and formulation consistency can be lacking. Melatonin has been used in dose ranges from 1 to 10 mg with benefits. Side effects can include headache, daytime sedation, increased dreaming, nausea, and hypothermia. Melatonin is generally not recommended for patients with dementia (Auger et al., 2015).

Nonpharmacological Treatment of Sleep Disorders

- Sleep hygiene
- Cognitive behavioral therapy—insomnia

Pharmacological Treatment of Sleep Disorders

- Antidepressants
- Histamine receptors
- Melatonin receptors
- Benzodiazepines
- Nonbenzodiazepine hypnotics

An 82-year-old Caucasian male, Mr. W, presents to his psychiatric provider with a chief complaint of "I can't sleep," and requests a prescription for a "sleeping pill." Mr. W presents to the office alone but ambulates with the assistance of a three-prong walker. He appears frail and walks with a noticeable curvature of the spine, stooped over and with an uneven gait.

Mr. W is pleasant and responds appropriately to questions regarding possible mood symptoms. His responses are appropriate to topic, and he appears to not have any deficits related to hearing or cognition. He denies any persistent difficulty with depressed mood, daytime anxiety, or issues with psychotic symptoms. His discussion perseverates upon his inability to stay asleep, which has been ongoing for the past couple of years but worsening to a daily problem over the past 6 to 9 months.

Typically, Mr. W wakes around 6 a.m., lays in bed for 30 minutes, and then dresses and performs his morning routine. His routine consists of dressing in his housecoat and slippers, walking to the front door from the bedroom of his one-story home to retrieve the newspaper, and making himself a piece of toast with butter and a cup of black coffee. He lives alone; however, his son or daughter, who both reside nearby, often come check in on him on their way to work in the mornings around 8 a.m. By this time, Mr. W is generally dressed, showered, and working in his garage on hobbies or performing tasks around the home. He requires assistance with heavy lifting, and his children often drive him on errands and to doctor's appointments, although he still maintains his driver's license. He may sit during the day and watch TV or read a newspaper for a few hours. He may typically nap one to two times per week for 30 minutes.

Mr. W's wife died 2 years ago after battling a terminal illness. He spent the previous 3 years providing around-the-clock care for his wife. She died at home peacefully. While caring for his wife, he would often be up several times per night giving her medication or attending to her needs. Since her death, he has reported more

(continued)

difficulty with sustaining sleep. He usually falls asleep within a half-hour of going to bed but wakes 2 hours later and cannot fall back asleep. Mr. W does admit to making frequent trips to the bathroom during the night but does not feel an urgency to urinate is waking him. He does not report severe nightmares, vivid dreams, or any significant problems with pain. In the morning, he sometimes may feel that he is still fatigued and as though he has not slept at all. However, he will wake at 6 a.m. without an alarm, usually, and start his day.

At this time, Mr. W has been self-medicating with diphenhydramine 25 mg as needed at bedtime for the management of his sleep complaints. He reports variable benefits from the diphenhydramine.

The patient has a history of hypertension, and his current medication is atenolol 50 mg/day. He also takes an OTC MVI, a calcium supplement, and fish oil. He does not have any dietary restrictions and drinks one to two cups of coffee in the mornings and one to two cups of herbal tea to soothe himself some evenings. He is a former smoker and quit 15 years ago after a 1 ppd smoking history. No current substance abuse or use. No reports of alcohol use.

PHYSICAL EXAM

Mr. W is healthy; his BMI is within normal limits. No abnormal breath sounds or heart sounds. He has a mild general weakness and an unsteady gait, especially without his walker. His blood pressure reads 148/86 mmHg and pulse is 68 bpm. He generally has an unremarkable physical exam.

Questions:

1. Based upon the limited patient history and current symptoms presented so far, what else might you want to ascertain about his history and symptoms? What other specific questions might you consider related to the patient's sleep?

2. After reviewing some of the rating scales available for use in your evaluation, please choose one and discuss why you are using this scale, what information it might provide for you, and what you expect the outcome to be.

(continued)

3. What are your thoughts about Mr. W's current use of diphenhydramine? Would you recommend the patient continue to use this medication?

4. What referrals would you make, if any?

Interprofessional Box

After evaluating Mr. Jeffers, a 65-year-old married male, you determine that he does not suffer from insomnia, hypersomnia, or narcolepsy. You believe he meets the criteria for obstructive sleep apnea (OSA) based upon the symptoms he and his wife describe during the evaluation. How would you best describe your findings to Mr. Jeffers and his wife in terms they can understand and to whom would you make a referral? What predisposing factors to OSA would you include in your description?

To best describe OSA to a patient, the provider should include a discussion about disrupted airway functioning during OSA. During sleep, patients will attempt to breathe normally; however, the airway becomes restricted or completely obstructed so that less oxygen is able to get through. Some typical clinical features of a patient with OSA include being obese, possible comorbid hypertension, complaints of snoring, awakening during the night feeling as though the patient cannot breathe, and daytime drowsiness and fatigue, to name a few. Patients should be referred to a sleep specialist or for a follow-up sleep study. During a sleep study, patients will be observed for abnormal EEG results and recorded for the number of apneic episodes that occur through the night according to polysomnography. According to the National Institute of Neurological Disorders and Stroke (NINDS), polysomnography measurements also typically include recording breathing rates, oxygen saturation, eye and limb movements, and heart rate (NINDS, 2019).

(continued)

An EEG uses small electrodes attached to the scalp to record brain activity, which looks like waves on output. The electrical activity can be measured and compared to expected brain activity during different stages of sleep. A sleep specialist may then determine whether a patient enters each phase of sleep and the duration.

Evidence-Based Practice Box

The primary initial recommendation for sleep disorders in geriatric patients is cognitive behavioral therapy for insomnia (CBT-I). CBT-I can consist of therapy through individual session, group therapy, or even web-designed or self-help texts. If medications are to be used, insomnia treatment guidelines often suggest using medications short term for no more than 4 to 5 weeks at a time (Qaseem et al., 2016).

CRITICAL THINKING QUESTION

When initially discussing sleep problems with a geriatric patient, prior to prescribing sleep medications, what criteria might you assess other than sleep quality and quantity to obtain a proper sleep history? If you determine sleep medication may be indicated, which medications are you least likely to consider first due to age?

REFERENCES

American Geriatrics Society Beers Criteria® Update Expert Panel. (2019). American Geriatrics Society 2019 Updated AGS Beers Criteria® for potentially inappropriate medication use in older adults. *Journal of the American Geriatrics Society*, *67*(4), 674–694. https://doi.org/10.1111/jgs.15767

Auger, R. R., Burgess, H. J., Emens, J. S., Deriv, L. V., Thomas, S. M., & Sharkey, K. M. (2015, October). Clinical Practice guideline for the treatment of intrinsic circadian rhythm sleep-wake disorders: Advanced sleep-wake phase disorder (ASWPD), delayed sleep-wake phase disorder (DSWPD), non-24-hour sleep-wake rhythm disorder (N24SWD), and irregular sleep-wake rhythm disorder (ISWRD). An update for 2015: An American Academy of Sleep Medicine Clinical Practice Guideline. *Journal of Clinical Sleep Medicine, 11*(10), 1199–1236. https://doi.org/10.5664/jcsm.5100

Buysse, D. J., Rush, A. J., & Reynolds, C. F. (2017, November 28). Clinical management of insomnia disorder. *Journal of the American Medical Association, 18*(20), 1973–1974. https://doi.org/10.1001/jama.2017.15683

Chen, L., & Yang, G. (2015, April). Recent advances in circadian rhythms in cardiovascular systems. *Frontiers in Pharmacology, 6,* 71. https://doi.org/10.3389/fphar.2015.00071

Foley, D. J., Monjan, A., Simonsick, E. M., Wallace, R. B., & Blazer, D. G. (1999). Incidence and remission of insomnia among elderly adults: An epidemiologic study of 6,800 persons over three years. *Sleep: Journal of Sleep Research & Sleep Medicine, 22*(Suppl. 2), S366–S372.

Kamel, N. S., & Gammack, J. K. (2006). Insomnia in the elderly: Cause, approach, and treatment. *American Journal of Medicine, 119*(6), 463–469. https://doi.org/10.1016/j.amjmed.2005.10.051

Mayo Clinic. (2019). *Obstructive sleep apnea.* https://www.mayoclinic.org/diseases-conditions/obstructive-sleep-apnea/diagnosis-treatment/drc-20352095

National Institute of Neurological Disorders and Stroke. (2019, August). *Brain basics: Understanding sleep.* https://www.ninds.nih.gov/Disorders/Patient-Caregiver-Education/Understanding-Sleep

Qaseem, A., Kansagara, D., Forciea, M. A., Cooke, M., Denberg, T. D.; Clinical Guidelines Committee of the American College of Physicians. (2019, July). Management of chronic insomnia disorder in adults: A clinical practice guideline from the American College of Physicians. *Annals of Internal Medicine, 165*(2), 125–133. https://doi .org/10.7326/M15-2175

Sateia, M. J., Buysse, D. J., Krystal, A. D., Neubauer, D. N., & Heald, J. L. (2017). Clinical practice guideline for the pharmacologic treatment of chronic insomnia in adults: An American Academy of Sleep Medicine Clinical Practice Guideline. *Journal of Clinical Sleep Medicine, 13*(2), 307–381. https://doi.org/10.5664/jcsm.6470

Stahl, S. M. (2017). *Prescriber's guide: Stahl's essential psychopharmacology* (6th ed.). Cambridge University Press.

Wennberg, A. M., Canham, S. L., Smith, M. T., & Spira, A. P. (2013, November). Optimizing sleep in older adults: Treating insomnia. *Maturitas, 76*(3), 1–10. https://doi .org/10.1016/j.maturitas.2013.05.007

CHAPTER 8

SUBSTANCE USE DISORDER IN GEROPSYCHIATRY

HELENE VOSSOS

DAVID J. MOKLER

LEARNING OBJECTIVES

After reviewing this chapter, practitioners will be able to:

- identify diagnostic criterion for substance use disorders
- analyze specific assessments for alcohol use disorder, benzo-diazepine use disorder, and opioid use disorder
- apply assessment tools and evaluate differential diagnoses to identify substance use disorders
- evaluate risks and comorbidities of geropsychiatric populations with substance use disorders
- understand treatment options for geropsychiatric populations with substance use disorders disorder

■ INTRODUCTION

In this chapter, practitioners will be introduced to substance use disorders in geropsychiatric populations, identifying criteria for diagnosis, assessments, and evaluating comorbidities, including differential diagnoses and indications for treatment options. This chapter will discuss the differences in addiction, dependence, tolerance, intoxication, substance withdrawal, and treatment options for geropsychiatric populations. A case study will be presented with differential diagnoses and risk factors for comorbidities. Substance use disorder assessment tools will be discussed including evidence-based treatment options.

■ PREVALENCE AND ETIOLOGY

Substance use disorders (SUD) affect more than 1 million older adults age 65 years or older in the United States, ("older adults"). Research suggests 978,000 (9%) older adults have an alcohol use disorder (AUD) and 161,000 have an illicit substance use disorder (American Psychiatric Association, 2013). In adults age 50 or older, illicit substance use is projected to increase from 2.2% to 3.1%, and alcohol use disorder is projected to increase from 2.8% to 5.7% over the next 10 years. This emergence is a public pandemic and rates are higher in illicit substance use disorders in the baby-boom generation (those born between 1946 and 1964) compared to prevalence in other generations (National Institute on Alcohol Abuse and Alcoholism, 2008).

Epidemiologic studies indicate, 6 million older adults drink an average of two drinks per day, measuring a minimum of 11 days per month of alcohol consumption. Research studies indicate 469,000 older adults consumed an illicit drug such as cannabis, cocaine (including crack cocaine), opioids (including heroin), hallucinogenics, inhalants, and sedatives or hypnotics (benzodiazepines) (Rhoads & Murphy, 2015). In older adults, alcohol use disorder is the number one SUD diagnosis related to hospital admissions or increased risk for death by age 60, and heroin or other opioids are the number one reason for emergency department visits, which equals to more than 1 million visits annually by older adult populations. Research revealed that other substances such as antidepressants or antipsychotics, in corroboration with an alcohol or illicit substance, accounted for 25% of emergency department visits (Mattson et al., 2017). This is a cause for concern as older adults with dual diagnoses such as depressive or mood disorders, generalized anxiety disorder, or previous trauma history are using alcohol and/or illicit substances at alarming rates (Searby, Maude, & McGrath, 2015). Incidence of alcohol and/or substance use in dual diagnosis older adults has grown and account for more than 50% of the cases.

■ DEFINITIONS

- Abuse (of substance): Use of a chemical substance or drug substance that deviates from the approved medical or social norms and patterns.

- Misuse: Use of a prescription that is not taken as prescribed.

- Intoxication: A reversible state caused by a specific chemical substance or drug substance that affects impairment in one or more of function, such as memory, orientation, mood, judgment, mental functioning, social functioning, behavioral functioning, or occupational functioning.

- Addiction: Repeatedly increasing and uncontrolled use of a substance despite adverse consequences.

- Dependence:

  ❏ Physical dependence: Repeated use of a chemical substance or drug that, on cessation, leads to specific withdrawal syndromes.

  ❏ Psychological dependence: Repeated use of a chemical substance or drug that, on cessation, leads to intense cravings and the risk of relapse.

- Dual diagnosis: Co-existence of a substance use disorder and a psychiatric disorder.

- Substance use disorder: An umbrella term for substance abuse and dependence.

- Tolerance: Repeated use of a chemical substance or drug that results in a decreased effect over time of repeated use, requiring larger amounts to be ingested to obtain the effect of the original dose.

- Withdrawal: A cluster of physiological and emotional symptoms that occur after stopping or reducing = substance use; may affect vital signs, physical signs and symptoms, thought process, emotions, and behaviors.

- Neuroadaptation: Occurs when there are neurochemical and/or neurophysiological changes to the body as a result of repeated use of the chemical or drug substance.

- Codependence: When family members or loved ones affected by substance users enable, allow, or facilitate their family member's use. This includes the family member becoming unwilling to accept the addiction as a mental health disorder and denying that the person is abusing substances.

■ DIAGNOSTIC CRITERION FOR SUBSTANCE USE DISORDER

The *Diagnostic and Statistical Manual*, Fifth Edition *(DSM-V)* outlines the diagnostic criteria for alcohol and substance use disorders (American Psychiatric Association, 2013). Hallmarks of these criteria are:

- uncontrolled use of the drug
- repeated attempts to cut down or quit
- a significant amount of time spent obtaining and using the drug
- cravings to use
- continued use despite adverse consequences
- use interferes with responsibilities at work or home
- tolerance and withdrawal
- Two or more of these need to occur over a 12-month period.

CASE 8.1

A 72-year-old female, "Mrs. B," presents to the clinic with a 40-year history of episodic binge alcohol consumption. Her chief complaint is, "I have been so anxious lately, my hands will not stop shaking."

PAST MENTAL HEALTH HISTORY

Mrs. B has had symptoms of anxiety, night sweats, hand tremors, occasional facial twitches, stomach cramps with occasional vomiting in the morning, headache, and labile blood pressure and tachycardia. She shares that she has always been a social drinker, but lately over the last year, "she has to drink in the morning so she will not shake or vomit." Her sister has given her some of her lorazepam to "stop the anxiety." She noticed "it stopped the handshakes, too," and she is requesting a prescription for lorazepam. She has never had any substance use treatment and denies her social binging with alcohol is a problem. She is hesitant to openly talk about her alcohol use, although today she is stating she fell last night and "needs an x-ray of her head."

Current and Past Psychotropic and Medical Medication History

Current medication list includes: Sertraline (Zoloft) 100 mg Q am (has taken it for 20 years), carvedilol 3.125 mg BID, lovastatin 40 mg at HS, aspirin 325 mg one to two tabs TID as needed for recurrent headaches. She has failed alprazolam, as her state data base showed at last visit that she was taking more than was prescribed; last prescription was 6 months ago.

Psychiatric Hospital History: Mrs. B was never in the inpatient psychiatric unit or the hospital other than for a caesarian section delivery.

(continued)

Social History: Mrs. B is widowed; she lives alone in an apartment complex in Savannah, Georgia. She had been married 45 years prior to becoming a widow. She has two children who live out west in California. She has a bachelor's degree in teaching and retired 9 years ago. She has a membership in the garden club but has not been attending functions for the past year. She has a history of two previous DUIs, which were over 5 years ago, and she has had her drivers licensed renewed this year. She denies any current legal charges related to substance or alcohol use.

Past Medical/Surgical History: Mrs. B has a history of hypertension, dyslipidemia, arthritis, major depressive disorder, generalized anxiety disorder, and tobacco use (50 pack per year history). She had a cesarean section at age 28, bilateral knee replacements at age 60, and only uses aspirin for pain.

SUBJECTIVE

She endorses her mood as anxious, lonely, and experiencing excessive worry since her fall. She reports she rates anxiety in the mornings 10/10, has symptoms of tremors and nausea, sometimes vomits with no real food in her stomach, sweats at night and sometimes in the morning, and noticed anxiety was less after she consumed three (8 ounce) glasses of red wine. When asked to take the CAGE assessment tool, she screened positive for alcohol use disorder. Her urine toxicology screen was positive for benzodiazepines and she admits she was taking someone else's lorazepam (Ativan). In quantifying her use further, she states she started drinking age 32 after she had her children, and was drinking socially at first with her spouse. She shares she would drink only on the weekends, although as her children moved away, she noticed she began drinking daily; every night she would consume three or four glasses of wine, drinking more on the weekends, until she reached 750 mL of red wine daily over the past 2 years. Her last drink was yesterday at night. She admits to taking lorazepam nightly "to fall asleep." She states she started taking them for her handshakes in the morning, but found they helped her go to sleep. She started to

(*continued*)

take lorazepam twice a day about 1.5 years ago, when "she could not handle the anxiety from the hand shakes, tremors, and anxiety" when she was running low on wine. She presents intoxicated, with the odor of alcohol on her breath.

MENTAL STATUS EXAM

Mrs. B appears with fair hygiene, mismatched clothing, fair eye contact, she reports her mood as anxious, and is objectively anxious with an intoxicated affect changing to a smiling affect incongruently. She is cooperative, with normal volume but slurred speech. Thought process is concrete and denial of substance and alcohol use is a problem. Thought content is linear to disorganized at times; she does not appear to be hallucinating. She denies suicidal thoughts but does indicate she would jump off a bridge if she could not get the anxiety or tremors to stop. Concentration is impaired. Remote memory is intact and recent memory is impaired, as she cannot state what she ate for meals today and is unable to complete the three item recall. Insight is poor, judgment is limited to impaired.

Initial laboratory data and vital signs: BP 166/102, HR 104, benzodiazepines in her initial urine toxicology results and breathalyzer alcohol level is 0.20.

Questions:

1. Based on the patient's history and current symptoms presented so far, how do you think you might proceed with assessment/evaluation questions and interview? What treatment could you recommend? Would you recommend outpatient or inpatient treatment?

2. After reviewing diagnostic criteria for substance use disorder and alcohol use disorder, what rating scales would you use to evaluate her condition? Please choose one and discuss why you are using that scale. What other evaluations could be beneficial for finding out what differential diagnosis list would be developed for analysis?

(continued)

3. What are your thoughts about her current mental status exam and urine toxicology results?

4. What release of information would you consider? What referrals or interprofessional treatment team members would you want to include for her treatment?

Differential Diagnoses

Differential diagnoses include other substance use disorders, mistreatment such as elder abuse (encompassing physical, emotional or sexual abuse), neglect, Korsakoff's syndrome or Wernicke's encephalopathy, and hepatic or metabolic encephalopathy (Sadock, Sadock, & Ruiz, 2015).

The practitioner will need to complete a full history and physical examination in addition to a mental status examination, drug urine toxicology screening with confirmatory serum toxicology laboratory analysis and blood alcohol level, and comprehensive laboratory panel that should include serology such as hepatitis series, rapid plasma reagent (RPR) to evaluate for syphilis, ammonia level to assess for hyperammonia, B12 and folate levels, and thyroid-stimulating hormone, as this full analysis will evaluate for medical etiologies (Sadock, Sadock, & Ruiz, 2015).

■ ASSESSMENT TOOLS

■ CAGE: Alcohol screening test (Exhibit 8.1)

■ Clinical Institute Withdrawal Assessment for Alcohol (CIWA-AR; Exhibit 8.2)

■ Clinical Opiate Withdrawal Scale (COWS; Exhibit 8.3)

EXHIBIT 8.1

CAGE ALCOHOL ASSESSMENT TOOL

CAGE QUESTIONNAIRE ASSESSMENT TOOL

1. Have you ever felt you should **C**ut down on alcohol?

2. Have people **A**nnoyed you by criticizing your drinking?

3. Have you ever felt bad or **G**uilty about your drinking?

4. Have you ever had a drink first thing in the morning (as an **E**ye-opener) to steady your nerves or get rid of a hangover?

Scoring: 2 or 3 strongly suggests a problem with alcohol

SOURCE: CAGE: Mayfield, D., McLeod, G., & Hall, P. (1974). *Essentials of psychiatric mental health nursing: Concepts of care in evidence-based practice* (6th ed., p. 310). (Cited by Townsend, M. [2014].)

EXHIBIT 8.2

CIWA-ASSESSMENT OF ALCOHOL WITHDRAWAL

Patient's Name: _____ Date: _____ Time: _____ Pulse or heart rate, taken for one minute:_____ Blood pressure: _____	
Nausea and vomiting. Ask "Do you feel sick to your stomach? Have you vomited?" Observation: 0———No nausea and no vomiting 1———Mild nausea with no vomiting 2———	**Tactile disturbances.** Ask "Do you have you any itching, pins-and-needles sensations, burning, or numbness, or do you feel like bugs are crawling on or under your skin?" Observation: 0———None

(continued)

3———

4———Intermittent nausea with dry heaves

5———

6———

7———Constant nausea, frequent dry heaves, and vomiting

Tremor. Ask patient to extend arms and spread fingers apart. Observation:

0———No tremor

1———Tremor not visible but can be felt, fingertip to fingertip

2———

3———

4———Moderate tremor with arms extended

5———

6———

7———Severe tremor, even with arms not extended

Paroxysmal sweats
Observation:

0———No sweat visible

1———Barely perceptible sweating; palms moist

2———

3———

4———Beads of sweat obvious on forehead

5———

6———

7———Drenching sweats

1———Very mild itching, pins-and-needles sensation, burning, numbness 2———Mild itching, pins-and needles sensation, burning, or numbness

3———Moderate itching, pins-and-needles sensation, burning, or numbness

4———Moderately severe hallucinations

5———Severe hallucinations

6———Extremely severe hallucinations

7———Continuous hallucinations

Auditory disturbances. Ask "Are you more aware of sounds around you? Are they harsh? Do they frighten you? Are you hearing anything that is disturbing to you? Are you hearing things you know are not there?" Observation:

0———Not present

1———Very mild harshness or ability to frighten

2———Mild harshness or ability to frighten

3———Moderate harshness or ability to frighten

4———Moderately severe hallucinations

(continued)

5——Severe hallucinations
6——Extremely severe hallucinations
7——Continuous hallucinations

Anxiety. Ask "Do you feel nervous?"
Observation:
0——No anxiety (at ease)
1——Mildly anxious
2——
3——
4——Moderately anxious or guarded, so anxiety is inferred
5——
6——
7——Equivalent to acute panic states as occur in severe delirium or acute schizophrenic reactions

Agitation
Observation:
0——Normal activity
1——Somewhat more than normal activity
2——
3——
4——Moderately fidgety and restless
5——
6——

Visual disturbances. Ask "Does the light appear to be too bright? Is its color different? Does it hurt your eyes? Are you seeing anything that is disturbing to you? Are you seeing things you know are not there?"
Observation:
0——Not present
1——Very mild sensitivity
2——Mild sensitivity
3——Moderate sensitivity
4——Moderately severe hallucinations
5——Severe hallucinations
6——Extremely severe hallucinations
7——Continuous hallucinations

Headache, fullness in head. Ask "Does your head feel different? Does it feel like there is a band around your head"
Do not rate for dizziness or lightheadedness; otherwise, rate severity.
0——Not present
1——Very mild
2——Mild
3——Moderate
4——Moderately severe
5——Severe
6——Very severe
7——Extremely severe

(continued)

7———Paces back and forth during most of the interview or constantly thrashes about	**Orientation and clouding of sensorium.** Ask "What day is this? Where are you? Who am I?" Observation: 0———Orientated and can do serial additions 1———Cannot do serial additions or is uncertain about date 2———Date disorientation by no more than two calendar days 3———Date disorientation by more than two calendar days 4———Disorientated for place and/or person Total score: _____ (maximum = 67) Rater's initials _____

SOURCE: Sullivan, J. T., Sykora, K., Schneiderman, J., Naranjo, C. A., & Sellers, E. M. (1989). Assessment of alcohol withdrawal: The revised clinical institute withdrawal assessment for alcohol scale (CIWAAr). *British Journal of Addiction, 84*(11), 1353–1357. Reproduced with permission from Wiley Online Library.

EXHIBIT 8.3

CLINICAL OPIATE WITHDRAWAL SCALE (COWS)

For each item, circle the number that best describes the patient's signs or symptoms. Rate on just the apparent relationship to opiate withdrawal. For example, if heart rate is increased because the patient was jogging just prior to assessment, the increased pulse rate would not add to the score.

Patient: _____ Date and Time: _____	
Reason for this assessment _____	
Resting Pulse Rate: _____ beats/minute *Measured after patient is sitting or lying for one minute* 0 pulse rate 80 or below 1 pulse rate 81 – 100 2 pulse rate 101 – 120 4 pulse rate greater than 120	**GI Upset:** *over last 1/2 hour* 0 no GI symptoms 1 stomach cramps 2 nausea or loose stool 3 vomiting or diarrhea 5 multiple episodes of diarrhea or vomiting
Sweating: *over past 1/2 hour not accounted for by room temperature or patient activity.* 0 no report of chills or flushing 1 subjective report of chills or flushing 2 flushed or observable moistness on face 3 beads of sweat on brow or face 4 sweat streaming off face	**Tremor** *observation of outstretched hands* 0 no tremor 1 tremor can be felt, but not observed 2 slight tremor observable 4 gross tremor or muscle twitching
Restlessness *Observation during assessment* 0 able to sit still 1 reports difficulty sitting still, but is able to do so 3 frequent shifting or extraneous movements of legs/arms 5 unable to sit still for more than a few seconds	**Yawning** *Observation during assessment* 0 no yawning 1 yawning once or twice during assessment 2 yawning three or more times during assessment 4 yawning several times/minute

(continued)

Pupil size	Anxiety or Irritability
0 pupils pinned or normal size for room light 1 pupils possibly larger than normal for room light 2 pupils moderately dilated 5 pupils so dilated that only the rim of the iris is visible	0 none 1 patient reports increasing irritability or anxiousness 2 patient obviously irritable or anxious 4 patient so irritable or anxious that participation in the assessment is difficult
Bone or Joint aches *If patient was having pain previously, only the additional component attributed to opiates withdrawal is scored* 0 not present 1 mild diffuse discomfort 2 patient reports severe diffuse aching of joints/muscles 4 patient is rubbing joints or muscles and is unable to sit still because of discomfort	**Gooseflesh skin** 0 skin is smooth 3 piloerrection of skin can be felt or hairs standing up on arms 5 prominent piloerrection
Runny nose or tearing *Not accounted for by cold symptoms or allergies* 0 not present 1 nasal stuffiness or unusually moist eyes 2 nose running or tearing 4 nose constantly running or tears streaming down cheeks	Total Score _____ The total score is the sum of all 11 items Initials of person completing assessment: _____

Score: 5- 1 2 = mild; 13-24 = moderate; 25-36 = moderately severe; more than 36 = severe withdrawal

This version may be copied and used clinically.

Journal of Psychoactive Drugs   Volume 35 (2), April - June 2003

SOURCE: Wesson, D. R., & Ling, W. (2003). The Clinical Opiate Withdrawal Scale (COWS). *J Psychoactive Drugs, 35*(2), 253–9.

Exhibits 8.4 through 8.7 provide summarized information regarding the neuroadaptive reward center of the brain (Exhibit 8.4), the natural reward center of the mammalian brain (Exhibit 8.5), the addictive influences of dopamine (Exhibit 8.6), and the importance of prevention and education regarding substance abuse (Exhibit 8.7).

EXHIBIT 8.4

THE NEUROADAPTIVE REWARD CENTER

- All addictive drugs and humanistic activities release varying amounts of dopamine into the nucleus accumbens.

- Activation of synaptic dopamine, norepinephrine, and serotonin occurs.

- The mesolimbic (reward) pathway releases dopamine that originates from the ventral tegmental area (VTA) responsible for pleasure:

  ❏ activates rewards

  ❏ compulsions

  ❏ perseverance

  ❏ connects to the serotonin pathway

- The serotonin pathway is responsible for emotional regulation:

  ❏ mood

  ❏ memory

  ❏ cognition

  ❏ sleep

EXHIBIT 8.5

NATURAL REWARD CENTER: THE MAMMALIAN BRAIN

- The mammalian brain needs natural rewards: food, water, reproduction, nurturing, and shelter.
- Humans feel pleasure and are rewarded with natural rewards.
- In addiction, humans have fluctuations in dopamine → are physiologically reinforced for repetitive addictive behavior.
- Physical dependence of the natural reward center can reinforce substance use.

EXHIBIT 8.6

ADDICTIVE INFLUENCES OF DOPAMINE

- Humans release varying amounts of dopamine into the nucleus accumbens.
- Stimulant drugs release (cocaine and methamphetamine) the most dopamine.
- Alcohol or heroin influence the brain's own opiate system (endorphins).
- The effects of the dopamine reward pathway are mediated by gamma-aminobutyric acid (GABA).
- In non-addictive individuals, GABA is under continuous inhibition (neurotransmitter in anxiety disorders).
- Reinforcing or conditioning the reward center causes euphoria and subsequent addiction.
- Experiencing withdrawal and cravings for drugs (such as cocaine and methamphetamine) can influence substance use/relapsing.

EXHIBIT 8.7

PREVENTION IS KEY

- Primary prevention starts in childhood with education and in older adults' routine assessment. Education is key.

  - Assess for drug and/or alcohol use, domestic violence, and underlying mental disorders.

- Secondary prevention

  - Assess for relapses.

  - Assess for mental disorders.

  - Refer for outpatient psychiatric services or maintenance programs to reduce risks.

- Relapse prevention

  - Specialized programs are best practice.

  - Older adults who have legitimate physical pain syndromes requiring opioid medication refer to experienced practitioners to monitor carefully.

  - Support groups

Risk Factors and Comorbidities for Geropsychiatric Population

The number one risk factor for geropsychiatric populations for substance use disorders is loneliness. Second is chronic pain that may cause impaired mobility or poor physical health, leading to social role changes and poor economic or social support, which may progress to poor self-care. Other risk factors include misdiagnosis of a substance use disorder, undiagnosed abuse such as neglect or emotional, financial, physical, or sexual abuse, which may be undetected for years.

According to research, the American Geriatric Society reports older adults age 50 or older may be taking up to 90% of medications inappropriately or may misuse them. Although the average age of dependence on drugs such as cannabis, cocaine, or other stimulants, benzodiazepines, or opioids is 25 years old to 40 years of age, substance abuse can start in high school if not earlier in adolescence. Late-life substance dependence occurs from the ages of 40 to 60. This has been implicated with many consequences and comorbid medical risks such as hepatic failure, cognitive impairment, coronary events, and psychiatric dual diagnosed mood disorders and risk for suicide (Trevisan, Boutros, Petrakis, & Krystal, 1998).

Chronic pain is a significant risk factor that contributes to significant amounts of morbidity in the older population. Treatment of chronic pain continues to be an emergent field. Widely published clinical research is clear; opiates are not a treatment option for chronic pain. In addition to the high risk of dependency, they are not clinically effective. Treatments that are effective are psychotherapy, cognitive behavioral therapy, physical therapy, relaxation, and meditation. As far as pharmacotherapy is concerned, antidepressants and drugs such as gabapentin remain the most effective.

Treatment Options

Treatment options are dependent on the screening, diagnosis, and assessment of the substance, psychosocial stressors, and dual diagnosed psychiatric disorder. For alcohol use disorder with withdrawals, opioid use disorder with withdrawals, and benzodiazepine use disorder with withdrawal, detoxification in a substance use treatment center is recommended secondary to potential for risk of withdrawal seizure and sometimes death from withdrawal seizure (Bayard, Mcintyre, Hill, & Woodside, 2004). Dual diagnosis treatment centers are available for treating dual diagnoses such as major depressive disorder and alcohol use disorder simultaneously. Brief interventions are selected after a screening tool such as the CAGE CIWA-AR and COWS is completed. Brief detoxification programs that are 1 to 2 weeks have increased risk for relapse. Full substance use disorder and dual diagnosis treatment programs that are 30 to 90 days long use 12-step principles and therapeutic communities report the highest success rate for remission. Medication-assisted treatment is the use of FDA-approved "whole" patient approaches for populations with opioid use disorder or alcohol use disorder. This treatment may include either buprenorphine, a detoxification or office-based treatment to prevent withdrawals; naltrexone, an office-based non-addictive opioid antagonist that blocks the effects of opioids or alcohol cravings and is a daily pill or monthly injection; or methadone, a clinic-based opioid agonist that does not block other substances (Miller & Lalithkumar, 2013).

Substance use disorders specifiers are classified mild (presence of two to three symptoms), moderate (presence of four to five symptoms), or severe (presence of six or more symptoms). Early remission is 3 months of sobriety from the substance, sustained remission is classified of a period of 12 months or longer of sobriety from the substance.

Discussion

Research suggests substance use is an emerging health concern in older adults and is expected to rise from approximately 3 million to close to 6 million by 2020. Cohort studies reveal there are higher rates in the baby boom population (1946–1964). Negative consequences include medical comorbidities, social and family stressors, and isolation for older adults, which poses a risk for suicide. In addition, there are growing risks for overdoses and unintentional deaths. Substance use treatment is growing in this population, as it was reported 14,230 admissions were of age 65 or older. The number one primary substance is alcohol (29%) compared to opioids (including heroin, 6%) and cocaine/stimulants (2%). According to Substance Abuse and Mental Health Services (SAMHSA) only 5% of older adults were referred for substance use disorder treatment by a healthcare provider, 17% were initiated by the individual recognizing they had a substance use disorder, 3% were referred by a substance use disorder provider, 4% by community organizations, and 10% by the criminal justice system (2012, reported in 2014). Across the SAMHSA datasets, alcohol emerged as the main health concern and is problematic for populations aged 65 years and older. It is even more important to assess, diagnose, and refer geropsychiatric populations, discuss treatment options with family members and caregivers, refer to substance use treatment centers and counseling, and treat underlying mood disorders accordingly.

Interprofessional Box

After evaluating the 72-year-old female, who presented to the clinic with a 40-year history of episodic binge alcohol consumption, anxiety, tremors, and blood alcohol breathalyzer level of 0.20 and benzodiazepines in her initial urine toxicology report; inpatient detoxification in the hospital is clinically indicated as there is an elevated risk for seizure and perhaps death. This case study is symptomatic for withdrawal. Seizures may occur in 5% of untreated alcohol withdrawal cases and rises when benzodiazepines use is positive; risk of a fatal seizure may occur 48 to 72 hours after last consumption of alcohol or benzodiazepine and is considered a medical emergency.
Consider:

- Alcoholic Anonymous
- Narcotic Anonymous
- Certified addiction professional (CAP) counselor
- Counselor in addiction therapy.
- Dual diagnosis substance use treatment centers
- Medical necessity for medical detoxification in the hospital
- Family members or sober support peers for support

Evidence-Based Practice Box

Geriatric populations are treated appropriately according to clinical presentation and severity, and especially according to the presenting risk of potential for serious outcomes such as withdrawal seizures, death, or suicide. Evidence based practice includes expeditious admission for detoxification, rehabilitation with interventions of pharmacotherapy, monitoring physiologic, and psychologic status. In addition, nonpharmacologic psychosocial therapeutics are imperative to use. For example, motivational psychotherapy. Evidence-based treatment is driven by the length of time a substance has been misused or consumed; the withdrawal symptoms, including tolerance and long-term dependence, may lead to intentional or unintentional overdose (Trevisan, Boutros, Petrakis, & Krystal, 1998).

Evidence-based interventions are aimed at treating the person in a holistic research-based detoxification approach and rehabilitation, including treating underlying dual diagnoses such as depressive or mood disorders, generalized anxiety disorders, substance-induced anxiety disorders, and undiagnosed post-traumatic stress disorders, as undiagnosed psychiatric disorders are more termed dual diagnoses (Searby, Maude, & McGrath, 2015).

First-line pharmacologic medications prescribed for alcohol or benzodiazepine withdrawals are benzodiazepine tapers to reduce the risk for withdrawal seizures; adjunctive medications to treat withdrawal symptoms such as anxiety, elevated blood pressure, heart rate, tremors, dehydration, mood disorders, potential electrolyte balances, folate and thiamine deficiencies; and anticonvulsant medications aimed at reducing risk of withdrawal seizures. Thiamine, folic acid, and electrolyte assessment and replacement are essential to reduce risks of Korsakoff's syndrome or Wernicke's encephalopathy (Miller & Lalithkumar, 2013).

First-line pharmacologic medications prescribed for opioid withdrawals are opioid buprenorphine or buprenorphine/

(continued)

naloxone tapers aimed to reduce the severe withdrawal symptoms of anxiety, agitation, vomiting, restlessness, sweating or diaphoresis, bone pain, and myalgia, along with adjunctive medications to treat additional withdrawal symptoms such as insomnia and restless legs, and improving nutritional deficiencies while promoting recovery from opioids.

For geropsychiatric populations who experience amphetamine, cocaine, or cannabis use disorder and/or withdrawals, it is of extreme importance to screen for comorbid alcohol or benzodiazepine use as this could have severe serious life or death implication. For geropsychiatric populations who experience amphetamine, cocaine, or cannabis use disorders, prompt referral to a certified addiction professional (CAP) counselor or counselor in an addiction therapy or substance use treatment inpatient or outpatient center is the standard of plan for treatment. Self-desire for treatment improves prognosis.

Nonpharmacologic or psychotherapeutic approaches are aimed at treating psychosocial stressors, building on motivation, improving self-awareness managing self-thoughts, and maintaining motivation while moving away from addiction into a recovery mindset. Promoting and regulating sleep hygiene and building a community of sober support is therapeutic.

CRITICAL THINKING QUESTIONS

1. When initially meeting a geriatric patient with a suspected substance use disorder, what preliminary assessment questions might you want to ask? Why would these questions be essential to your knowledge while developing a treatment plan for their substance use disorder?

2. How will you want to manage the patient? Will geropsychiatric patients require more vigilant screening for dual diagnoses and monitoring?

REFERENCES

American Psychiatric Association. (2013). *Diagnostic and statistical manual of mental disorder* (5th ed.). https://doi.org/10.1176/appi.books.9780890425596

Bayard, M., Mcintyre, J., Hill, K., & Woodside, J. (2004). Alcohol withdrawal. East Tennessee State University, James H. Quillen College of Medicine, Johnson City, Tennessee *American Family Physician. 69*(6): p. 1443–1450.

Mattson, M., Lipari, R., Hays, C., & VanHorn, S. (2017). *A day in the life of older adults: Substance use facts.* The Center for Behavioral Health Statistics and Quality: Substance Abuse and Mental Health Services Administration (SAMHSA). https://www.samhsa.gov/data/sites/default/files/report_2792/ShortReport-2792.html

Miller, M. & Lalithkumar, S. (2013). Geriatric psychiatry. *Pittsburgh Pocket Psychiatry.* Oxford University Press: NY. p. 208–209.

National Institute on Alcohol Abuse and Alcoholism (2008). National Institute of Health. OMB# 0925-06482021. Accessed via the web: https://pubs.niaaa.nih.gov/publications/AlcoholFacts%26Stats/AlcoholFacts%26Stats.htm

Rhoads, J. & Murphy, P. (2015). Clinical consult to psychiatric nursing for advanced practice. Substance use disorders.

Sadock, B.J., Sadock, V.A. & Ruiz, P. (2015). Kaplan & Sadock's Synopsis of Psychiatry (11th Ed.). Philadelphia, PA: Wolters-Kluwer.

Searby, A., Maude, P., McGrath, I. (2015). Dual diagnosis in older adults: A review. *Issues in Mental Health Nursing.* 2/36. p. 104–111.

Trevisan, L., Boutros, N., Petrakis, I., Krystal, J. (1998). Complications of alcohol withdrawal: Pathophysiological insights. *Alcohol Health and Research World.* (22/1) p. 1–66.

CHAPTER 9

NEUROCOGNITIVE DISORDERS

WILLIAM S. SUTTON

After reviewing this chapter, practitioners will be able to:

- identify basic neurological changes in the geriatric client
- discuss screening tools that can be used to establish a neuro-cognitive disorder diagnosis
- define major and mild neurocognitive disorder (previously referred to as dementia in *DSM-IV*)
- identify neurocognitive disorder subtypes
- discuss basic etiology of neurocognitive disorder subtypes
- identify and assess patients for symptoms corresponding to neurocognitive disorders
- demonstrate basic understanding of pseudodementia
- recommend general pharmacological and non-pharmacological interventions for neuropsychiatric symptoms related-to neurocognitive disorders

■ INTRODUCTION

Roughly 47 million individuals live with major and mild neurocognitive disorders (NCDs) worldwide. Prevalence of NCDs is estimated to increase to 131.5 million by 2050 (Prince, 2015). In the United States, 5% and 20% of people over the ages of 65 and 80, respectively, have NCDs. Socioeconomic and cultural factors affect the rates of NCDs globally (Nepal et al., 2017).

NCDs are characterized by cognitive and functional impairment that develops over time. Changes include impairment to cognition, memory, language, and visuospatial functioning. Most NCDs are progressive (Agronin, 2015) and uncurable (Hugo & Ganguli, 2014). Concurrent behavioral disturbances and mood disorders occur in some people as well. NCDs are generally organized by subtype. Subtypes are characterized by duration of disease progression, functional domains affected, and symptomatology. NCDs with advanced age are commonly associated with degenerative central nervous system (CNS) disease as well as cardiovascular disease (Sadock et al., 2015). Obtaining a thorough medical history is crucial as proper diagnosis of an NCD subtype may depend on an underlying, somatic disease state (American Psychiatric Association, 2013).

The *DSM-V* and assessment scales area used in the diagnosis of NCDs. Neuropsychological and neurological testing can also be utilized to identify NCDs syndromes. These assessment tools include, but are not limited to, the Mini-Mental State Exam (MMSE), the Montreal Cognitive Assessment (MoCA), and the six-item cognitive impairment test (6-CIT). Lastly, both non-pharmacological and pharmacological therapies are available in managing cognitive, mood, and behavioral symptoms related to NCDs. These topics will be discussed at the end of this chapter.

■ NORMAL AGING

Biological changes, including those in brain physiology and memory, occur with advancing age. Tissue atrophy, the presence of white matter lesions, small vessel changes, and ventricle enlargement are some examples of normal brain aging (Guo et al., 2017). Such changes cause additive effects on cognition. Neurological studies including the use of MRI are used to objectively assess such changes. (Guo et al., 2017).

Many older adults report memory lapses that are commonly referred to as "senior moments." Memory lapses are common across the lifespan but appear to occur more frequently as an individual ages. Mental processing speed and sensory perception decline with normal aging. Such decline includes hearing loss as well as decreases in speech discrimination and sound localization (Murman, 2015). Evidence illustrates a decline in executive functioning skills, which include decision-making and problem-solving, with normal aging. Episodic memory, which accounts for one's autobiographical information, remains stable in the aging patient. However, new learning can be impaired with normal aging (Murman, 2015). Despite being bothersome, normal aging changes do not impair daily functioning. Many elderly peoples utilize lists, memory games, and memory training to improve daily life.

■ DIAGNOSTIC SCALES

There are various assessment scales used in the assessment and diagnosis of mild and major NCDs. Some, including the Mini-Cog and the 6-CIT, are suitable for primary care screening for NCD. Commonly used scales will be reviewed below. More specific and thorough cognitive testing is generally completed by neuropsychologists. Should this be needed, the APRN should refer the patient appropriately. Additionally, depression is common with neurocognitive disorder and assessment can be challenging in those with cognitive impairment. Common screening tools include the Geriatric Depression Scale (GDS), the Cornell Scale for depression in dementia, and the Montgomery-Asberg Depression Rating Scale (MADRS).

■ Mini-Cog

The Mini-Cog (Borson et al., 2003) is a short screening testing commonly completed in primary care settings. It can be completed in roughly 3 minutes. (Sheehan, 2012). It is a two-part test utilized to assess cognitive impairment. A patient is asked to remember three items and is then asked to remember them. Then, after drawing a clock, they are asked to recall the three items (Davis et al., 2013). According to Sheehan (2012), the Mini-Cog has a sensitivity of 76% and a specificity of 89%.

■ 6-CIT

The 6-CIT (Brooke & Bullock, 1999), Six-Item Cognitive Impairment Test, was designed for screening by the primary care clinician. It takes roughly 3 to 4 minutes to complete. It is utilized in the clinical diagnosis of dementia. The 6-CIT yields high sensitivity at 90% and specificity, 100%, respectively (Sheehan, 2012).

■ MMSE

The Mini-Mental State Exam (MMSE), is widely used and well known in clinical settings. IT takes around 10 minutes to complete by clinicians and assess cognitive function including orientation, memory, attention and calculation, and language and visual construction (Sheehan, 2012). It is a 30-question inventory used primarily as a screening test. It has modest sensitivity at 79%. There is research stating that the MMSE is psychometrically inferior to the SLUMS exam (Buckingham et al., 2013).

■ MoCA

The Montreal Cognitive Assessment (MOCA) was originally developed for the screening of mild cognitive impairment (mild NCD; Sheehan, 2012). It is a 30-item inventory that can be completed in 10 minutes. The test assesses short-term memory, executive functioning, attention, concentration and working memory, language, orientation, and visuospatial functioning (Davis et al., 2013). It is particularly useful for patients with vascular impairment, including vascular neurocognitive disorder (VND). The MOCA has high specificity at 100% and a specificity of 87% (Sheehan, 2012).

■ SLUMS

The Saint Louis University Mental Status (SLUMS) exam is a 30-point inventory designed to measure orientation, executive function, memory, and attention. The SLUMS is a sensitive screening tool that may be psychometrically superior to other screening tools in detecting cognitive impairments (Buckingham et al., 2013). The SLUMS exam includes animal naming and clock drawing, resulting in a thorough executive function assessment. This may explain this inventory's high sensitivity in identifying mild NCD (MCI; Howland et al., 2016).

■ RISK FACTORS FOR BOTH MILD AND MAJOR NEUROCOGNITIVE DISORDERS

Risk factors for mild and major NCDs vary regarding their etiological subtype. Old age is the strongest risk factor for NCD. This is in part due the increased risk of neurodegenerative and cardiovascular disease with age. More specifically, higher degrees of vascular and white matter changes in adulthood can increase one's risk of developing NCD with advanced age (Guo et al., 2017). Higher prevalence of NCDs, particularly NCD due to Alzheimer's disease (AD), is connected to female gender. This may be due to greater longevity in women (American Psychiatric Association, 2013). Other risk factors are related to lifestyle. Modifiable risk factors associated with increased risk of NCD diagnosis include history of mid-life obesity, hyperlipidemia, obesity, tobacco use, caffeine use, traumatic brain injury (TBI), depression, and sleep disturbances (Nepal et al., 2017).

■ MILD NEUROCOGNITIVE DISORDER

When a person experiences cognitive decline that exceeds that of normal aging, they are diagnosed with a mild neurocognitive disorder (Agronin, 2015). This disorder is frequently called mild cognitive impairment (MCI). Roughly 10% to 20% of individuals over the age of 65 are diagnosed with a mild NCD. Mild NCD represents the transition between normal aging and major MCD. Mild NCD is a broad diagnosis that is further characterized by the underlying disease etiology. Neurological changes of mild NCD include atrophy of medial temporal lobar brain regions, including the hippocampus and entorhinal regions, and posterior cingulate cortex. The temporal lobe is responsible for mediating conscious or declarative memory (Anderson, 2019). More specific cerebral changes are related to the degenerative disease etiology.

According to the *DSM-V* (American Psychiatric Association, 2013), diagnostic criteria include evidence of modest cognitive decline from previous performance level in one or more cognitive domains, including complex attention, executive function, learning and memory, language, perceptual-motor, or social cognition. Such decline is based on the concern of the individual, a knowledgeable informant, or clinician that cognitive decline is evident, as well as a modest impairment in cognitive performance. Such impairment may be documented by formal neuropsychological testing or another quantitative clinical assessment. The recognized cognitive deficits do not interfere with one's capacity to complete everyday activities, including paying bills and managing medications. In addition, the cognitive deficits do not occur exclusively in the context of a delirium or are not better explained by another mental disorder (American Psychiatric Association, 2013). Lastly, the clinician specifies whether the mild NCD is due to a given etiology such as Alzheimer's disease or frontotemporal lobar degeneration. Should etiology be unclear, the advanced practice registered nurse (APRN) lists the diagnosis as mild NCD, unspecified. It is important to note that a mild NCD may be due to multiple etiologies (American Psychiatric Association, 2013).

■ MAJOR NEUROCOGNITIVE DISORDER

Major NCDs represent a continuance in cognitive decline in one or more cognitive domains. Receiving a major NCD diagnosis indicates the progression of the underlying disease process responsible for cognitive and functional decline. As with mild NCD, major NCD is a broad term utilized to encompass various degenerative etiologies. The underlying pathology of major NCD is associated with specific disease subtypes (American Psychiatric Association, 2013). These subtypes include but are not limited to: NCD due to Alzheimer's disease, NCD due to Lewy body disease, NCD due to vascular neurocognitive disease, and NCD due to frontotemporal lobar degeneration. Other major NCDs are associated with medical conditions such as Parkinson's disease, TBI, HIV-infection, and prion disease (Agronin, 2015). This chapter highlights four NCDs commonly seen in practice.

According to the *DSM-V* (American Psychiatric Association, 2013), major NCD diagnostic criteria includes evidence of significant cognitive decline from an individual's previous level of performance in two or more cognitive domains, including complex attention, executive function, learning and memory, language, perceptual-motor, or social cognition. This is based on the concern of the individual, of a knowledgeable informant, or of the clinician that a significant decline in cognitive function has occurred. Evidence of cognitive decline is also based on substantial impairment in cognitive performance. This is documented through neuropsychological testing or another quantified clinical assessment. Additionally, one's cognitive deficits interfere with independence in daily living and activities such as paying bills or managing medications. Furthermore, cognitive deficits do not occur in the context of delirium and cannot be better explained by another mental disorder. Lastly, the clinician specifies the major NCD's etiological subtype. Should etiology be unclear, the advanced practice registered nurse (APRN) lists the diagnosis as mild NCD, unspecified. It is important to note that a major NCD may be due to multiple etiologies (American Psychiatric Association, 2013).

■ NEUROCOGNITIVE DISORDER DUE TO ALZHEIMER'S DISEASE

Major NCD due to Alzheimer's disease (AD), frequently referred to as "Alzheimer's disease (AD)", is the most common neurodegenerative disease (Hugo & Ganguli, 2014). AD is the sixth leading cause of death in the United States (Kirova et al., 2015). Depending on the clinical setting and use of diagnostic criteria, major NCD due to AD accounts for between 60% and 90% of major NCDs (American Psychiatric Association, 2013). Both mild and major NCD due to AD progress gradually through severe NCD and death. Cognitive decline is insidious in onset and progresses gradually and steadily (Hugo & Ganguli, 2014). AD typically presents during the eighth or ninth decades of life. However, early-onset AD can be diagnosed during the fifth decade of life. Prognosis is roughly 10 years after onset of NCD due to AD diagnosis. Most individuals with NCD due to AD die as the result of aspiration. Late-stage individuals are generally mute, bedbound, and require total care (American Psychiatric Association, 2013). The strongest risk factor for AD is advanced age (American Psychiatric Association, 2013).

AD is characterized by the progressive loss of neurons and synapses, cortical atrophy, the accumulation of amyloid plaques, and the presence of tau-predominant neurofibrillary tangles (American Psychiatric Association). Both plaques and tangles present within areas of the brain responsible for episodic memory, including medial temporal lobe structures (Kirova et al., 2015). Prominent cholinergic deficits are a hallmark of AD, as well. PET scans are commonly used to assess for amyloid deposition in the brain. In addition, MRI brain scans can present evidence of neuronal injury, including hippocampal atrophy (Hugo & Ganguli, 2014). A diagnosis of probable AD can be given based on family history and presence of genetic mutation through genetic testing (American Psychiatric Association, 2013).

Those with mild NCD appear to develop major NCD due to AD more rapidly than those without mild NCD. This may be due to the presence of beta-amyloid plaques and neurofibrillary tau tangles in mild NCD (Kirova et al., 2015). However, some mild NCD cases progress to non-AD dementias (Peterson & Negash, 2008).

In early AD, patients present with a progressive decline in learning and in memory. (American Psychiatric Association, 2013). Executive functioning is also impaired. Impairments and decline in visuoconstruction, perceptual-motor functions, language, and social cognition occur in the late-stage disease state (Hugo & Ganguli, 2014). Individuals may present with apathy and depression at any point through disease progression. In mild to late-stage AD, psychosis, irritability, agitation, wandering behaviors, and combativeness may be present. In late stage, gait disturbances, dysphagia, and incontinence may be present (Hugo & Ganguli, 2014).

Symptoms and diagnostic criteria are highlighted in the *DSM-V*. An individual is diagnosed with either probable of possible AD. To be diagnosed with NCD due to AD, an individual must meet criteria for either major or mild NCD. Disease presentation must be insidious in onset as well as a gradual progression of impairment in one or more cognitive domains. Criteria for probable major NCD due to AD include either evidence of a causative AD genetic mutation from family history or genetic testing, as well as evidence of decline in memory and learning in at least one cognitive domain; steadily progressive, gradual decline in cognition; and no evidence of mixed etiology. Should these criteria not be met, possible major NCD due to AD should be diagnosed. Lastly, the cognitive disturbances are not better explained by cerebrovascular disease, another neurodegenerative disease, effects of substance, or another mental, neurological, or systemic disorder. This same criterion is utilized to diagnosed probable or possible mild NCD due to AD. (American Psychiatric Association, 2013).

Treatment of NCD due to AD is focused on reduction of disease risk factors as opposed to treating the illness itself (Agronin, 2015). Further treatment is based on symptom management, particularly neuropsychiatric symptoms. These symptoms include psychosis, agitation, aggression, anxiety, sleep/wake disturbances, and apathy. Additionally, those with mild NCD with concurrent depressive symptoms progress to AD at a higher rate than those without (Lyketsos et al., 2011). Nonpharmacological interventions including exercise, environmental triggers, and use of music with bathing, as well as pharmacological interventions including antidepressant and antipsychotic medications, are used in treating mood, psychotic, and behavioral symptoms (Lyketsos et al., 2011). Use of acetylcholinesterase inhibitors (AChEI) is based on the hypothesis that cholinergic deficits occur with AD. Their use is associated with improvement and/or stabilization of cognition and functional abilities for a period of 10 to 12 months. Glutamate receptor antagonists may be used as well, as excitotoxic and abnormal glutamate transmission can injure and kill neurons (Agronin, 2015).

■ VASCULAR NEUROCOGNITIVE DISORDER

Major or mild vascular neurocognitive disorder (VND), also known as vascular dementia, is the second most common form of neurocognitive disorder (O'Brien & Thomas, 2015). Prevalence estimates for the United States range from 0.2% in those aged 65 to 70 years of age to 16% of individuals over the age of 80. Additionally, 20% to 30% of patients are diagnosed with NVD within the 3 months following stroke. Prevalence is higher in African American populations compared to Caucasians. It is seen more often in males (American Psychiatric Association, 2013).

The cognitive deficits related to VND are largely attributed to cerebrovascular disease. It is commonly present in conjunction with NCD due to AD. It results from both large and small vessel disease (Hugo & Ganguli, 2014). Proper diagnosis is based on history of stroke of transient ischemic attacks. Unfortunately, there are no clear pathological, diagnostic criteria as VND represents pathological changes (O'Brien & Thomas, 2015).

Clinical features of VND vary and are dependent on the location of lesions. Symptom presentation and prognostic timeline are variable as well (Hugo & Ganguli, 2014). Cognitive decline, particularly in areas of complex attention and executive functions, is common. Personality and mood changes and emotional lability are also frequently noted(American Psychiatric Association, 2013). VND-related depression is also seen in later life. Lastly, physical deficits including gait disturbances and urinary symptoms are also associated with VND (Hugo & Ganguli, 2014).

Risk factors include increasing age, low education, and multiple vascular risk factors (O'Brien & Thompson, 2015). Furthermore, risk factors associated with cerebrovascular disease, including diabetes, hypertension, smoking, and obesity, are the same as those for NVD (American Psychiatric Association).

According to the *DSM-V* (American Psychiatric Association, 2013), criteria for either major or mild NCD must be met in order to be diagnosed with VND. Clinical features must be consistent with vascular etiology as evidenced by either: the onset of the cognitive deficits is temporally related to one or more cerebrovascular events *or* the evidence for decline is prominent in complex attention and frontal-executive function. Additionally, evidence of the presence of cerebrovascular disease from history, physical examination, and/or neuroimaging considered enough to account for the neurocognitive deficits must be evident. Lastly, the symptoms cannot be better explained by another neurological disease or systemic disorder (American Psychiatric Association, 2013).

There are no pharmacological interventions with regulatory approval for the prevention and treatment of vascular dementia. There is research, however, that early treatment of hypertension appears to reduce the risk of VND. AChEI drugs as well as memantine may be beneficial on cognitive symptoms related to VND (Baskys & Cheng, 2012). The APRN should encourage use of nonpharmacological intervention in behavioral and mood management, such as music therapy, as well. Lastly, as previously mentioned, mood changes, including depression, are seen in late-stage VND. Treatment of these symptoms may be necessary.

■ NEUROCOGNITIVE DISORDER WITH LEWY BODIES

Neurocognitive disorder with Lewy bodies, formerly referred to as dementia with Lewy bodies, is prevalent in 0.1% to 5% of the general elderly population. Further estimates share that NCD with LB accounts for 1.7% to 30.5% of all NCD cases. Additionally, pathological lesions, referred to as Lewy bodies, are present in upwards of 35% of NCD cases. NCD with LB is more commonly diagnosed in men (American Psychiatric Association, 2013). Some studies suggest that NCD with LB may be more common than that of vascular neurocognitive disorder (VND; Agronin, 2015).

NCD with LB should not be confused with "Lewy body dementia" as Lewy body dementia is an umbrella term that includes the diagnoses of both NCD with LB (dementia with Lewy bodies) and NCD due to Parkinson's disease (Parkinson's disease dementia). Additionally, the use of "Lewy body disease" is a pathological, postmortem diagnosis based on the presence of Lewy body pathology upon physical examination (Armstrong, 2019). The division of neurocognitive disorder with LB and neurocognitive disorder due to Parkinson's disease (PD) is present in the *DSM* and are listed as separate diagnoses (American Psychiatric Association, 2103).

Lewy bodies, first discovered by Frederick Lewy in 1912, are intracytoplasmic, abnormal deposits of alpha-synuclein and ubiquitin proteins. Pathological features of NCD with LB include not only the presence of LB in subcortical and cortical areas of the brain, but also cerebral atrophy and beta-amyloid plaques, as seen with NCD due to AD (Agronin, 2015). A major neurological difference between NCD with LB and NCD due to AD is relative preservation of medial temporal lobes. Despite differences in initial clinical presentation, many symptoms of both NCD due to LB and NCD due to PD are similar as both illnesses show similar neurological changes upon autopsy (Gomperts, 2016).

Risk factors for NCD with LB include psychiatric history significant for anxiety and depression. In addition, those with NCD with LB are more likely to have a history of stroke, the presence of APOE ε4 alleles, and a family history of Parkinson's disease (PD). Individuals with NCD with LB tend to be younger than those with AD and are more likely to be male. Social risk factors include low rates of alcohol and caffeine use as well as being more educated (Boot et al., 2013).

Clinical features of NCD with LB include cognitive decline, severe sensitivity to neuroleptic medications, postural instability, falls, episodes of syncope or unresponsiveness, autonomic dysfunction, excessive daytime sleepiness, parkinsonian motor symptoms, delusions, visual hallucinations, apathy, anxiety, and depression (Armstrong, 2019). Early manifestation of rapid eye movement (REM) sleep behavior disorder is common as well (American Psychiatric Association, 2013). NCD due to PD exhibits similar symptomatology, including presence of hallucinations, parkinsonian motor symptoms, and cognitive dysfunction (Gomperts, 2016). A major distinction between NCD with LB and NCD due to PD is the time of onset of both motor and cognitive symptoms. In NCD with LB, cognitive dysfunction presents prior to parkinsonian motor symptoms. A diagnosis of NCD due to PD is warranted when cognitive decline occurs with well-established PD diagnosis. Cognitive decline begins early in those with NCD with LB, around age 55. Delusions are less common in NCD due to PD. Additionally, visual hallucinations are reportedly less fearful than those in NCD with LB. (Gomperts, 2016).

As with other neurocognitive disorders, a thorough history is crucial in proper NCD with Lewy bodies diagnosis. Thorough diagnostic testing is helping in the diagnosis of NCD with Lewy bodies (Gomperts, 2016). In addition to presence of clinical features explained above, SPECT or PET scans can be utilized to identify indicative biomarkers, including reduced basal ganglia dopamine transporter uptake (Armstrong, 2019). A supportive biomarker includes preservation of medical temporal lobe structure upon CT/MRI (Armstrong, 2019).

Per the *DSM-V*, diagnosis of NCD with LB includes diagnosis of mild or major MCD. The onset of symptoms must be insidious and indicate gradual progression. Core diagnostic features include fluctuating cognition with variations in attention and alertness; recurrent, well-formed visual hallucinations; and spontaneous parkinsonian features with subsequent onset following cognitive decline. Suggestive diagnostic features include meeting criteria for rapid eye movement sleep behavior disorder and severe neuroleptic sensitivity. Probable diagnosis is based on inclusion of two core diagnostic features, or one suggestive feature with one or more core features. Possible NCD with LB diagnosis is based on the presence of only one core feature or one more suggestive feature. Lastly, symptomatology cannot be better explained by cerebrovascular disease, other neurodegenerative disease, substance use, or other mental, neurological, or systemic disorder (American Psychiatric Association, 2013).

There is no curative treatment for NCD with LB. The APRN should focus on the improvement of psychosis, mood symptoms, and behavioral disturbances. A multidisciplinary approach to symptom management is important. Family education, particularly one's increased risk of neuroleptic sensitivity, is also vital (Agronin, 2015). Both acetylcholinesterase inhibitors (AChEI) and NMDA receptor antagonist medications may be used for cognitive impairment in those with NCD with LB. AChEI may also be helpful in improving psychomotor slowing, psychosis, and apathy. SSRI and SNRI medications can be used to treat a disease-related anxiety, depression, and apathy. Low dose antipsychotic/neuroleptic medication, such as quetiapine, can be utilized in the management of psychosis. However, it is of importance to recall that those with NCD with LB are sensitive to treatment with neuroleptics due to dopamine cell loss (Gomperts, 2016). Lastly, caregivers of those with NCD with LB are particularly burdened by behavioral disturbances and that are not managed well with medications. Nonpharmacological interventions in the management of behavioral disturbances including environmental adaptations, caregiver training, family education, and other behavioral strategies (Barton et al., 2016).

■ FRONTOTEMPORAL NEUROCOGNITIVE DISORDER

Major or mild frontotemporal neurocognitive disorder (FND), also referred to as frontotemporal dementia or Pick's disease, is a common type of NCD affecting approximately 20% to 50% of people under the age of 65 with NCD (Cardarelli et al., 2010).

FND is considered the third most prevalent dementia, with prevalence ranging from 3% to 26% of neurocognitive disorders (Bang et al., 2015). FND can mimic many psychiatric disorders due to its prominent behavioral features. Due to this, diagnosis is not only challenging, but often goes undiagnosed (Bang et al., 2015).

FND is characterized by atrophy of the frontal and temporal lobes. This disease is comprised of several syndromes characterized by progressive development of behavioral, personality, and or language impairment (Hugo & Ganguli, 2014). There are two identified variants of FND: the *behavioral variant* and the *language variant* (American Psychiatric Association, 2013). Disease presentation is insidious in onset and progresses gradually. Areas of brain atrophy correspond to underlying disease variance. Behavioral and language disturbances occur early on in disease state (Agronin, 2015). As FND progresses, symptoms related to clinical variants may converge (Bang et al., 2015). Prognosis illustrates survival 6 to 11 years after symptom presentation and 3 to 4 years following diagnosis (American Psychiatric Association, 2013). Death is typically caused by pneumonia or other secondary infection (Bang et al., 2015).

Etiology behind FND is largely unknown (Cardarelli et al., 2010). However, genetic factors have been identified, which include microtubule, gene encoding mutations associated with the tau protein, granulin gene, and the C9 (cC9ORF72) gene. Additionally, roughly 40% of individuals with diagnosed FD have a family history significant for early-onset NCD. Familial transition of the disease is possible (American Psychiatric Association, 2013). Genetic predisposition appears to be an important risk factor for FND (Band et al., 2018). Lastly, pre- and postsynaptic changes in serotonin occur in FND, which may be associated with behavioral changes and disorders of the disease (Barton et al., 2016).

Disease and clinical presentation depend closely on syndromic variant identified. Those individuals with behavioral-variant FND present with degrees of apathy or disinhibition. This apathy is at times misdiagnosed as depression (Cardarello et al., 2010).

In addition, individuals may lack interest in socialization, self-care, and personal responsibilities. Some may display inappropriate social behavior. Cognitive deficits are less prominent in early disease states. Although impairment in executive function is impaired in many, learning and memory may be preserved (American Psychiatric Association, 2013).

Language-variant FND presents with gradual onset of progressive aphasia. Subtypes of language-variant, progressive aphasia FND include semantic variant, agrammatic/non-fluent variant, and logopenic variant. Each have their own unique presentations corresponding to underlying neuropathology (American Psychiatric Association, 2013). Semantic-variant FND presents with anomia for people, places, and objects. Word-finding difficulties and word comprehension are evident. As this disease variant progresses, behavioral and affective changes occur (Bang et al., 2015). Non-fluent variant FND is characterized by slow, labored, halting speech production as well as agrammatism. Individuals may have difficulty understanding sentence with complex syntax structure. Mild anomia may be present (Bang et al., 2015). Logopenic patients may be distinguished by lack of speech sound distortions and syntactic errors. Speech rate differs from that of both semantic and non-fluent variants as well (Henry & Gorno-Tempini, 2010). Over time, patients present with global cognitive decline. Motor deficits, including parkinsonism and motor neuron disease, may be present as well (Bang et al., 2015).

Diagnosis of FND requires a thorough examination including history and family history. Insidious disease onset and relative preservation of memory are important in differentiating FND from other NCDs, such as NCD due to AD. Neuroimaging including MRI and neuropsychological testing are helpful in FND diagnosis (Cardarello et al., 2010). Per the *DSM-V* (American Psychiatric Association, 2013), criteria for either major or mild NCD must be met for diagnosis of FND. Second, patient presentation must have insidious onset and gradual symptom progression. The behavioral variant is diagnosed with presence of three or more of the following behavioral symptoms: behavioral disinhibition; apathy or inertia; loss of sympathy or empathy; perseverative, stereotyped or compulsive ritualistic behaviors; hyperorality; and dietary changes. Prominent decline in social cognition and/or executive abilities must also be present. The language variant is diagnosed with presence of prominent declining in language ability in the form of speech production, word finding, object naming, grammar, or work comprehension. Relative sparing of learning and memory, as well as perceptual-motor function, must be exhibited as well. Lastly, the individual's presentation and associated disturbances cannot be better explained by cerebrovascular disease, another neurodegenerative disease, or another mental, neurological, or systemic disorder (American Psychiatric Association, 2013).

There is no cure for FND. Symptom management and family-centered care are hallmarks of treatment. Psychotropics can be utilized for symptom management (Cardarello et al., 2010). Selective serotonin reuptake inhibitors (SSRI) may be beneficial for behavioral symptoms, depressive symptoms, and inappropriate behaviors. Aggressive behaviors or outbursts may respond well to low-dose antipsychotics. The roll of acetylcholinesterase inhibitors (AChEI) is unclear as patients with FND have persevered cholinergic function. Galantamine, however, may be helpful in those with non-fluent aphasia (Cardarello et al., 2010). Nonpharmacologic interventions include addressing caregiver needs and functional issues. Reducing noise and stimulation and simplifying social situations are helpful to those with FND. Addressing sensory needs that one may not be able to verbalize is also encouraged. Music therapy may also be of therapeutic value (Barton et al., 2016).

■ OTHER SUBTYPES

The four common forms of mild and major NCD are reviewed above. Other etiological subtypes are outlined in the *DSM-V* and are seen in clinical practice. Each possible etiology is medical or substance-induced in nature. Some examples include NCD due to traumatic brain injury, NCD due to HIV infection, and NCD due to Huntington's disease. Each diagnosis has a common structure. First an individual must meet criteria for either mild or major neurocognitive disorder. Then, the substance-induced or medical etiology must be established while excluding other causes (Sachdev et al., 2014). Each diagnosis has its own risk and prognostic factors, diagnostic markers, and treatment guidelines (American Psychiatric Association, 2013). Diagnostic criteria and information for each NCD subtype can be found in the *DSM-V*.

■ PSEUDODEMENTIA

Pseudodementia (PDEM) is a clinical state, resembling dementia (NCD), occurring concurrently with an underlying psychiatric disorder (Dua & Grover, 2018). PDEM is commonly used to describe the cognitive deficits in many psychiatric disorders, particularly geriatric depression (Kang et al., 2014). These patients are often misdiagnosed and treated for NCD when the underlying disorder, for example, depression, goes untreated (Dua & Grover, 2018). Severe cognitive impairment due to depression can cause confusion between diagnosing NCD versus depression. It is important to note that both NCD and depression can co-exist (Kang et al., 2014).

There are diagnostic features that assist the APRN in differentiating between PDEM and NCD. A key component of PDEM is its reversibility. Cognition improves with proper treatment of the underlying psychiatric condition. In contrast, many NCDs are irreversible. PDEM is associated with rapid onset and progression. NCD progresses gradually and is insidious in onset. Those presenting with PDEM are more likely to have a psychiatric history compared to those with NCD. Individuals with pseudodementia can provide subjective information and share distress as it relates to the cognitive deficits. Lastly, PDWM presents with consistent, depressed mood, whereas mood symptoms fluctuate in those with NCD (Dua & Grover, 2018).

CASE 9.1

Mr. Edward Jones is a 72-year-old married Caucasian male with no significant psychiatric history. He is well-spoken and highly educated. Mr. Jones presents to your outpatient, primary care office at the recommendation of his son, Patrick. The patient's son suggested to his father that he receives a "check-up" as he has been increasingly more forgetful over the last 2 months. He has a history of well-controlled hypertension for which he is prescribed metoprolol and amlodipine. There are no recent reports of falls, head trauma, or loss of consciousness. There is no history of cognitive deficits prior to 2 months ago.

Mr. Jones lives with his wife, who suffers from chronic pain and requires assistance with activities of daily living. He is her primary support. Edward reports recent change in motivation in caring for his wife and that energy is "lacking." They are visited by Patrick weekly. Edward is a retired high school history teacher who worked until the age of 68, when he chose to retire. Mr. Jones worked for "all of his life" and has joked that he would never retire as he had a passion for teaching. Over the past few months, Edward has not attended a poker group in which he participates with friends. He endorses intermittent sadness and not wanting to read the newspaper due to poor concentration. He corroborates his son's claims that he has been more forgetful. Mr. Jones can describe his symptoms and feels that he is having difficulty caring for his wife due to his memory. He is concerned and feels that he has dementia.

Questions:

1. Which neuropsychiatric symptoms are present in Mr. Jones's history? What clinical inventory or scale can be used in his evaluation?

(continued)

2. Mr. Jones and is concerned about his cognitive changes. Is the patient's presentation consistent with a neurocognitive disorder or pseudodementia?

3. What is/are Mr. Jones's diagnosis/diagnoses?

4. Is Mr. Jones on medications that can cause mood symptoms?

5. Discuss appropriate treatment options for Mr. Jones.

Interprofessional Box

The APRN administers the Mini-Cog screening assessment in the primary care office. Understanding the link between cognitive impairment and depression, the APRN also administers the Geriatric Depression Rating Scale. Edward scores a "3" on the mini-cog, accurately completing the clock drawing but forgettsing two of the words he was asked to remember. A score of three indicates lower likelihood of neurocognitive disorder but does not rule out cognitive impairment (Borson et al., 2003). Additionally, Mr. Jones scores a nine on the Geriatric Depression Rating Scale indicative of depression (Yesavage, 1988). The adult geriatric APRN refers Mr. Jones to a local psychiatric mental health APRN who diagnoses Mr. Jones with major depressive disorder, most likely due to lack of fulfillment following retirement and stress of caring for his wife. He is started on an SSRI medication, escitalopram. In addition, Mr. Jones is referred to a therapist to help treat his depressive symptoms. Lastly, Edward is presented with information regarding the use of a clinical social worker who may be able to provide both assistance and referrals in caring for his wife.

After 6 weeks, not only did Mr. Jones's mood improve, but his cognition improved as well. His presentation is not only consistent with major depression, but also pseudodementia.

■ CONCLUSION

By 2050, prevalence of NCDs is estimated to increase to 131.5 million (Prince, 2015). With that said, 5% and 20% of persons in the United States over the age of 65 and 80, respectively, currently have NCDs. The APRN will be responsible for assessing and managing neurocognitive disorders and their related symptomatology. The four most common types of neurocognitive disorders were reviewed in this chapter. However, other etiological subtypes of neurocognitive disorders exist. Obtaining a thorough assessment and history is vital in the screening of patients for neurocognitive disorders. Various diagnostic screening tools are available for the APRN in primary care settings. Further and more specific screening can be completed with the psychiatric mental health APRN, a neuropsychologist, or other medical providers trained in the assessment of neurocognitive disorders upon referral from the adult geriatric APRN. Neuropsychiatric disorders and symptoms, including depression, are common co-occurring illnesses in those with neurocognitive disorders. Assessment of both cognitive symptoms and mood symptoms is important for the accurate diagnosing of the geriatric client. Lastly, both nonpharmacological and pharmacological interventions are available for the treatment of mood and behavioral symptoms commonly associated with neurocognitive disorders. Interventions should be tailored to each specific neurocognitive disorder.

REFERENCES

Agronin, M. E. (2015). The dementia caregiver: A guide to caring for someone with alzheimer's disease and other neurocognitive disorders. Lanham, MD: Rowman & Littlefield.

American Psychiatric Association. (2013). *Diagnostic and statistical manual of mental disorder* (5th ed.). https://doi.org/10.1176/appi.books.9780890425596

Anderson, N. (2019). State of the science on mild cognitive impairment (MCI). *CNS Spectrums, 24*(1), 78–87. https://doi.org/10.1017/S1092852918001347

Armstrong, M. J. (2019). Lewy body dementias. *Continuum: Lifelong Learning in Neurology, 25*(1), 128–146. https://doi.org/10.1212/01.CON.0000532159.43885.85

Bang, J., Spina, S., & Miller, B. L. (2015). Frontotemporal dementia. *Lancet (London, England), 386*(10004), 1672–1682. https://doi.org/10.1016/S0140-6736(15)00461-4

Barton, C., Ketelle, R., Merrilees, J., & Miller, B. (2016). Non-pharmacological management of behavioral symptoms in frontotemporal and other dementias. *Current Neurology and Neuroscience Reports, 16*(2), 14. https://doi.org/10.1007/s11910-015-0618-1

Baskys, A., & Cheng, J. X. (2012). Pharmacological prevention and treatment of vascular dementia: Approaches and perspectives. *Experimental Gerontology, 47*(11), 887–891. https://doi.org/10.4103/0972-2327.132613

Boot, B. P., Orr, C. F., Ahlskog, J. E., Ferman, T. J., Roberts, R., Pankratz, V. S., Dickson, D. W., Parisi, J., Aakre, J. A., Geda, Y. E., Knopman, D. S., Petersen, R. C., & Boeve, B. F. (2013). Risk factors for dementia with Lewy bodies: A case-control study. *Neurology, 81*(9), 833–840. https://doi.org/10.1212/WNL.0b013e3182a2cbd1

Borson, S., Scanlan, J. M., Chen, P., & Ganguli, M. (2003). The Mini-Cog as a screen for dementia: Validation in a population-based sample. *Journal of the American Geriatrics Society, 51*(10), 1451–1454. https://doi.org/10.1046/j.1532-5415.2003.51465.x.

Brooke, P., & Bullock, R. (1999). Validation of a 6 item cognitive impairment test with a view to primary care usage. *International Journal of Geriatric Psychiatry, 14*(11), 936–940.

Buckingham, D. N., Mackor, K. M., Miller, R. M., Pullam, N. N., Molloy, K. N., Grigsby, C. C., . . . & Winningham, R. G. (2013). Comparing the cognitive screening tools: MMSE and SLUMS. *Pure Insights, 2*(3), 1–7.

Cardarelli, R., Kertesz, A., & Knebl, J. A. (2010). Frontotemporal dementia: A review for primary care physicians. *American Family Physician, 82*(11), 1372–1377. https://www.aafp.org/afp

Davis, D. H., Creavin, S. T., Noel-Storr, A., Quinn, T. J., Smailagic, N., Hyde, C., Brayne, C., McShane, R., & Cullum, S. (2013). Neuropsychological tests for the diagnosis of Alzheimer's disease dementia and other dementias: A generic protocol for cross-sectional and delayed-verification studies. *The Cochrane Database of Systematic Reviews*, (3), CD010460. https://doi.org/10.1002/14651858.CD010460

Dua, D., & Grover, S. (2018). Don't forget me: Pseudodementia associated with depression. *Journal of Geriatric Mental Health, 5*(2), 159. https://doi.org/10.4103/jgmh.jgmh_29_18

Gomperts, S. N. (2016). Lewy body dementias: Dementia with Lewy bodies and Parkinson Disease dementia. *Continuum, 22*(2 Dementia), 435–463. https://doi.org/10.1212/CON.0000000000000309

Guo, H., Siu, W., D'Arcy, R. C., Black, S. E., Grajauskas, L. A., Singh, S., Zhang, Y., Rockwood, K., & Song, X. (2017). MRI assessment of whole-brain structural changes in aging. *Clinical Interventions in Aging, 12*, 1251–1270. https://doi.org/10.2147/CIA.S139515

Henry, M. L., & Gorno-Tempini, M. L. (2010). The logopenic variant of primary progressive aphasia. *Current Opinion in Neurology, 23*(6), 633–637. https://doi.org/10.1097/WCO.0b013e32833fb93e

Howland, M., Tatsuoka, C., Smyth, K. A., & Sajatovic, M. (2016). Detecting change over time: A comparison of the SLUMS examination and the MMSE in older adults at risk for cognitive decline. *CNS Neuroscience & Therapeutics, 22*(5), 413–419. https://doi.org/10.1111/cns.12515

Hugo, J., & Ganguli, M. (2014). Dementia and cognitive impairment: Epidemiology, diagnosis, and treatment. *Clinics in Geriatric Medicine, 30*(3), 421–442. https://doi.org/10.1016/j.cger.2014.04.001

Kang, H., Zhao, F., You, L., Giorgetta, C. D., V., Sarkhel, S., & Prakash, R. (2014). Pseudo-dementia: A neuropsychological review. *Annals of Indian Academy of Neurology, 17*(2), 147–154. https://doi.org/10.4103/0972-2327.132613

Kirova, A. M., Bays, R. B., & Lagalwar, S. (2015). Working memory and executive function decline across normal aging, mild cognitive impairment, and Alzheimer's disease. *BioMed Research International,* 2015, 1–24. https://doi.org/10.1155/2015/748212

Lyketsos, C. G., Carrillo, M. C., Ryan, J. M., Khachaturian, A. S., Trzepacz, P., Amatniek, J., Cedarbaum, J., Brashear, R., & Miller, D. S. (2011). Neuropsychiatric symptoms in Alzheimer's disease. *Alzheimer's & Dementia, 7*(5), 532–539. https://doi.org/10.1016/j.jalz.2011.05.2410

Murman, D. L. (2015). The impact of age on cognition. *Seminars in Hearing, 36*(3), 111–121. https://doi.org/10.1055/s-0035-1555115

Nepal, H., Jeffrey, B., & Bhattarai, M. (2017). Dementia: Risk factors and updated review. *Journal of Psychiatrists' Association of Nepal, 6*(2), 3–7. https://doi.org/10.3126/jpan.v6i2.21750

O'Brien, J., & Thomas, A. (2015). Vascular dementia. *The Lancet, 386*(10004), 1698–1706.

Petersen, R. C., & Negash, S. (2008). Mild cognitive impairment: An overview. *CNS spectrums, 13*(1), 45–53.

Prince, M. J. (2015). *World Alzheimer Report 2015: The global impact of dementia: An analysis of prevalence, incidence, cost and trends.* Alzheimer's Disease International. https://www.alz.co.uk/research/WorldAlzheimerReport2015.pdf

Sachdev, P. S., Blacker, D., Blazer, D. G., Ganguli, M., Jeste, D. V., Paulsen, J. S., & Petersen, R. C. (2014). Classifying neurocognitive disorders: The *DSM-5* approach. *Nature Reviews Neurology, 10*(11), 634. https://doi.org/10.1038/nrneurol.2014.181

Sadock, B. J. Sadock, V. A. & Ruiz, P. (2015). Synopsis of psychiatry: Behavioral sciences clinical psychiatry (11th ed). New York: Wolters Kluwer.

Yesavage, J. A. (1988). Geriatric depression scale. *Psychopharmacol Bull*, *24*(4), 709–711.

CHAPTER 10

SEXUAL DYSFUNCTION IN THE OLDER ADULT

MATTHEW KEESLAR
ALAN W. SKIPPER
JOANNE ZANETOS

LEARNING OBJECTIVES

After reviewing this chapter, practitioners will be able to:

- define sexuality and sexual dysfunction
- distinguish differences in impotence and erectile dysfunction
- explain the hormonal changes in aging adult women
- apply principles of interdisciplinary collaboration to clinical practice
- identify risk factors for genito-pelvic pain/penetration disorder, orgasmic disorder, and female sexual interest/arousal disorder
- recommend evidence-based practice interventions to older adults suffering from reproductive changes
- establish a differential for erectile dysfunction in the aging male
- explain options for medical management and treatment of erectile dysfunction
- describe how age itself can be a risk factor for sexual dysfunction in the aging male
- describe how cardiovascular disease and diabetes can contribute to erectile dysfunction

■ INTRODUCTION

As patients grow older, the incidence of sexual dysfunction increases while sexual activity decreases. Multiple factors contribute to sexual problems, and older age compounds and complicates those factors. Although sexual activity can diminish with age, it helps to acknowledge that more than half of older adults are sexually active (Morton, 2017). Further, the majority of men and women over the age of 65 reports an interest in sex. Even with their interest in sex and increased sexual dysfunction, a minority of respondents to sexual activity studies reported talking to a healthcare provider about sex and sexuality since the age of 50 (Morton, 2017).

■ SEXUAL DYSFUNCTION IN THE AGED MALE

Aging alters male sexuality physiology. On average, it requires more time and more stimulation to become sexually aroused. A decrease in elastic fibers in the fascia of the penis, the tunica albuginea, results in less firm erections. Ejaculatory volume and force of ejaculation typically diminish. Detumescence is more immediate and the refractory period is longer (Morton, 2017). With all of these changes, however, the most prevalent sexual disorder in the aging male is erectile dysfunction (ED).

Erectile Dysfunction

Erectile dysfunction (ED) is the inability to achieve or maintain an erection sufficient for penetrative sexual activity. Studies consistently illustrate the prevalence of ED increasing with age (O'Donnell et al., 2004). In a landmark research effort, the Massachusetts Male Aging Study (MMAS) demonstrated that among the 1,709 men enrolled, 52% of those aged 40 to 70 years had ED symptoms (O'Donnell et al., 2004). The prevalence of some degree of ED increased by roughly 10% each decade past the age of 50. Further, men in their 60s reported ED symptoms four times more often than men in their 40s (O'Donnell et al., 2004). By tracking older men over a 17-year period, the MMAS showed the importance of age as a risk for sexual dysfunction in men.

While age itself poses a risk, an astute clinician will consider the myriad other conditions that contribute to ED. From a psychiatric perspective, the investigation of erectile dysfunction in the aging male begins by examining iatrogenic etiologies because psychopharmacology can contribute to sexual dysfunction (Liang et al., 2012). Additionally, many iatrogenic causes become evident when reviewing the patient's history. Polypharmacy, for example, is common in older adults (Maher et al., 2014) and can contribute to sexual dysfunction. Competing treatments and adverse effects of multiple medications may worsen ED (Gareri et al., 2014) or complicate diagnosis and treatment.

Further, medications used to treat depression and other psychiatric conditions are correlated to erectile dysfunction (Yafi et al., 2016). Although there is a clear risk of psychogenic erectile dysfunction in patients presenting to a mental health provider, many of the medications used to treat these patients may also add to the etiology. Patients treated for depression report a fivefold increase in complete ED, which exceeds the risk of ED attributed to depression itself (Francis et al., 2007). First-generation antipsychotics tend to worsen ED (Gareri et al., 2014). Medications for anxiety, Parkinson's, and bipolar mood disorder have all been shown to negatively impact sexual function (Gareri et al., 2014). Thus, the psychiatric provider must weigh the efficacy of the treatment for psychiatric disorders against possible increases in sexual dysfunction in the older male.

The psychiatric practitioner may also discover past genitourinary surgery or trauma on review of history, both of which significantly contribute to the risk of ED. Pelvic surgery, pelvic trauma, and spinal cord injuries can all disrupt the nerves necessary for erection and penile sensation (Dean & Lue, 2005). Radical prostatectomy for prostate cancer is perhaps the most significant iatrogenic contribution to ED in the aging male, even with the advent of nerve-sparing procedures. Other pelvic surgery for cancer or trauma can significantly impact erectile function as can trauma itself (Sangkum et al, 2015). A careful review of the patient history helps illuminate iatrogenic etiologies of ED in the aging male that can contribute to psychogenic causes.

■ ERECTILE DYSFUNCTION IN THE AGING MALE

ED can be a symptom of many other disorders related to aging. The differential for ED is extensive and the psychological component is significant. It is important, however, to consider other etiologies. Those etiologies typically falls into one of five categories that may be remembered as the mnemonic VANES: vascular, anatomic, neurologic, endocrinologic, and systemic disease.

■ VASCULAR CHANGES

Vascular disorders are the most common conditions causing erectile dysfunction in the aging male (Yafi et al., 2016). The hemodynamics of erections require adequate blood flow to the penis and then adequate trapping of blood in the corpora (Figure 10.1). Multiple studies have shown an increase in vasculogenic ED in patients with many common disorders associated with older patients, including:

1. Hypertension and patients treated with hypertension medication.

2. Dyslipidemia: elevated total and low-density lipoprotein cholesterol are more common in men with moderate to severe ED.

3. Diabetes: ED is a common condition in older men with diabetes and patients presenting with ED may have previously undiagnosed diabetes.

(Burnett et al., 2018; Francis et al., 2007; Yafi et al., 2016)

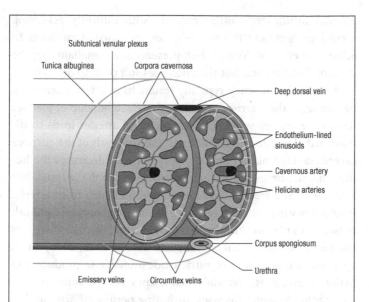

FIGURE 10.1 Diagrammatic cross-section of penis. As pictured here, the penis is basically three tubes. The corpora cavernosa on dorsal side is covered by a specialized fascial layer, the tunica albuginea. The cavernosa are cylinders that fill with blood to form an erection. On the ventral side, the corpus spongiosum surrounds the urethra. During an erection, the corporal arteries deliver blood to the sinusoids via the helicine arteries. Blood returns to the venous system via the emissary veins to the circumflex veins in the subtunical venular plexus. The expanding sinusoids and the tunica itself compress the outgoing veins, trapping blood inside the cavernosa.

The vascular insults associated with the above conditions may be grouped into two general classes: arterial insufficiency and venous leak. Arterial dysfunction implies decreased blood flow from the heart and can inhibit oxygenation of the erectile tissues.

Arterial insufficiency often presents with difficulty achieving a rigid erection and the necessity for increased stimulation to achieve an erection. Venous leak presents as a compliant that the erection first hardens, but then becomes soft prior to orgasm.

Arterial insufficiency typically results from arteriosclerosis, a hardening of the arteries, or atherosclerosis, a buildup of plaques within the arterial walls. The narrowing of arteries leads to diminished blood flow to the arteries and sinusoids of the corpora cavernosa. Diminished blood supply not only decreases the hemodynamics necessary to build pressure inside the corpora, but also starves the erectile tissue of oxygen. Ischemia from arterial insufficiency may ultimately lead to replacement of penile smooth muscle with fibrous connective tissue. Further, vascular disease is connected to endothelial dysfunction (Aversa et al., 2010) and a decrease in the amount of nitric oxide available to produce and maintain erections. Arterial insufficiency can be connected to many other vascular diseases, including peripheral arterial disease and tobacco use disorder. Further, ED is itself an independent risk factor for cardiovascular disease (Burnett et al., 2018).

Venous leak typically presents as an inability to maintain an erection. In normal erections, emissary veins from the corpora are compressed by the expanding sinusoids (Figure 10.1). As men age, the number and size of venous outflow paths increase (Morton 2017). With the resultant distension of the subtunical venular plexus, the expanding sinusoids of the corpora can no longer compress outflowing veins. Diminished ability to trap blood in the sinusoids causes the blood pressure in the cavernosa to drop; the cavernosa cannot sustain tumescence and the erection recedes (Figure 10.2).

■ ANATOMICAL CHANGES

Normal penile anatomy promotes firm erections. Peyronie's disease (PD), which is analogous to an arthritis of the penis, is a buildup of fibrous tissue in the tunica. Although we do not know exactly what causes PD, we do know that the prevalence increases

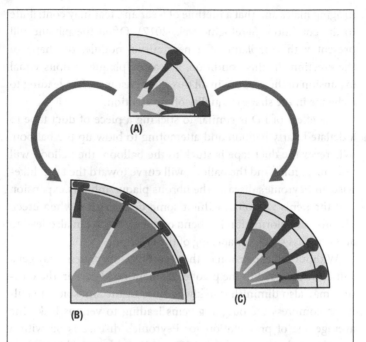

(A)

(B)

(C)

FIGURE 10.2 Diagrammatic explanation of venous leak in the aging male.

A. In the flaccid penis, the sinusoids are not distended and the blood flows back through the venous system without obstruction.

B. In a healthy erection, the sinusoids distend and compress the outgoing venous plexus between the sinusoids and the tunica.

C. In the aging male, there is an increase in venous outflow tracks along with an inflexible tunica that renders the sinusoids incapable of compressing the outgoing venous plexus, letting the trapped blood slowly leak back into venous circulation.

in aging males and that a lifetime of wear and tear may contribute to the condition (Serefoglu et al., 2017). Often the patient will present with complaint of a new curve, nodule, or shape of the erection. In this condition, a scar or plaque inhibits equal expansion of the corpora in all three dimensions, often leading to a change in the shape or quality of the erection.

The effect of PD is similar to sticking a piece of duct tape to a deflated party balloon and attempting to blow up the balloon. Wherever the duct tape is stuck to the balloon, the balloon will not inflate fully, and the balloon will curve toward the tape. Likewise, in Peyronie's disease, the fibrous plaque inhibits expansion and the penis will often exhibit some deformation when erect. Usually the deformation is a bend or curve, but it can also lead to an hourglass shape or tapering of the erection.

Without full expansion of the cavernosa, the patient may get a soft erection distal to the plaque. As mentioned earlier, the erection may also diminish quickly because of the sinusoids' inability to compress the outgoing veins leading to venous leak. The average age of presentation for Peyronie's disease is 55 with a prevalence that ranges from 0.4% to 13%, although this is likely an underestimation due to lack of reporting (Nehra et al., 2015). Although there are other anatomical abnormalities that can cause erectile dysfunction, Peyronie's disease remains a relatively common condition among older men.

■ NEUROLOGIC DISORDERS

Peripheral or central neurologic disease is another common cause of ED in the aging male. The neurology of erections can be classified into three types: central, autonomic, and peripheral. Centrally stimulated, or psychogenic, erections originate in the brain with sexual thoughts, visual and auditory sensations (Dean & Lue, 2005). Erections at the autonomic level are stimulated by the parasympathetic nervous system and require the non-adrenergic, non-cholinergic neurotransmitter nitric oxide (Dean & Lue, 2005). Finally, the peripheral somatic nerve input from the sacral nerve plexus contributes to reflexogenic erectile function. Reflexogenic erections require the tactile stimulation of the genital organs (Dean & Lue, 2005) and are diminished in neuropathies that diminish somatosensory input. A limitation in any of these neural pathways can contribute to erectile dysfunction.

Neuropathology can effect erectile function on many levels. Cerebrovascular accident, Parkinson's, and depression can alter central nerve processing. Diabetes and other neuropathies can impair sensation as well as autonomic efferent nerve signaling. Pelvic nerve damage from surgery or injury can also cause ED (Sangkum et al., 2015). Men who have had radical prostatectomies, for example, will often have a period of erectile dysfunction that can last up to a year, even with nerve sparing surgeries. Studies have shown that early medical intervention for patients undergoing prostatectomy can improve recovery and prevent fibrosis of erectile tissues (Dean & Lue, 2005). Thus, peripheral neuropathies due to aging, along with many higher brain disorders that affect older men such as Alzheimer's, multiple sclerosis, and cerebrovascular insufficiency, can also have a significant impact on erectile dysfunction.

■ ENDOCRINE DISORDERS

Many studies have illustrated the prevalence of andropause, or decline in male sex hormones with age. Low testosterone can indeed lead to lower libido, difficulty achieving erections, and decreased penile sensation (Morton, 2017). Further, direct-to-consumer advertising has heightened patients' awareness of testosterone deficiency and testosterone replacement therapy. Cross-sectional studies have shown a yearly decline of about 1% in men over the age of 30 (O'Donnell et al., 2006). Unfortunately, testosterone replacement without any other intervention has had little success as a treatment for ED in older men. Still, responsiveness to PDE5 inhibitors like Viagra does increase when androgen levels are within the normal range (Hwang et al., 2006).

Other endocrine disorders may also contribute to ED. Endocrinopathy has been estimated to account for 5% to 35% of erectile dysfunction. Hyperprolactinemia is associated with ED, lower libido, and decreased ejaculate volume (Nimbi et al., 2020). Both hyper- and hypothyroidism are associated with ED and decreased libido (Carson et al., 1999). Diabetes represents a significant risk factor for ED and the risk increases with age. Twice as many men with diabetes over the age of 65 report erectile dysfunction when compared with the average population; the prevalence of ED in diabetic patients ranges from 20% to 85%, with higher prevalence in patients with increased duration of diabetes (Burnett et al., 2018). Endocrine disorders that affect the hypothalamic-pituitary gonadal axis and contribute to systemic disease can contribute significantly to sexual dysfunction in the aging male.

■ SYSTEMIC ILLNESS

As mentioned above, diabetes mellitus has a significant impact on erectile function, but many other systemic illnesses can also alter sexual function. In this way, erectile dysfunction can be thought of as a bellwether responding to various affronts to whole organ systems. Smoking, for example, not only leads to COPD and decreased oxygenation of tissues, but also decreased blood supply to the cavernosa due to changes in vascular tonicity (Biebel et al., 2016). Alcoholism can decrease testosterone by contributing to liver disease but can also contribute to neurologic dysfunction. Hypertension and hypertension treatments also significantly increase the likelihood of erectile dysfunction. Thiazide diuretics and beta-blockers are two classes of antihypertensive that are strongly associated with ED.[7] Sexual dysfunction in the aging male is also strongly associated with metabolic syndrome (Schulster et al., 2017) and its associated disorders such as central obesity and hyperlipidemia. As systemic illnesses compound over a lifetime, so too do the risks for ED.

History

Some details of the history of erectile dysfunction help point the practitioner to etiologies other than psychogenic causes. For example, if the erectile dysfunction is equally prominent with both a partner and with masturbation, or if there is a complete absence of nocturnal erections, there may be further medical factors contributing to ED. Rapid onset of ED could indicate psychogenic cause but could also be attributed to recent genitourinary trauma or surgery. Sexual dysfunction contributes to low libido, but so does testosterone deficiency (Nimbi et al., 2020). It is also important to distinguish erectile dysfunction from premature ejaculation or inability to penetrate due to prominent curvature of the penis. Asking about medications, alcohol, and tobacco use can point the psychiatric provider to comorbid etiologies of ED.

Treatment

Current AUA guidelines recommend shared decision-making when considering treatment in the patient presenting with erectile dysfunction (Burnett et al., 2018). Discussing the treatments available in a straightforward manner with clear language helps improve patient autonomy and allows a collaboration between the patient and provider. This partnership helps determine the testing and treatment modalities best suited to the patient. The provider should first counsel patients on comorbidities that increase the likelihood of ED, diet and exercise, cardiac risk, and the need for follow-up with a primary care provider (PCP). The patient should be counseled on limiting alcohol, quitting smoking and street drugs, and decreasing stress. Along with psychiatric counseling, there are four modalities for helping men achieve better erections based on health history and contraindications.

1. Oral medications (PDE5 inhibitors): Medications such as sildenafil, tadalafil, and vardenafil can be used each day to help with erectile function. These phosphodiesterase

inhibitors should not be taken with anti-anginal nitrates such as isosorbide or nitroglycerin. They all work by increasing blood flow to the penis when the patient is sexually aroused. They all require sexual stimulation and should be taken about an hour before sexual activity on an empty stomach.

2. Vacuum erectile device: This is a pump that is placed over the penis and causes a vacuum that increases flow of blood to the cavernosa. Once an erection has been achieved, a constriction band can be placed over the penis to hold the erection while the man has sexual activity. The vacuum erectile device can be used with the oral medications.

3. Injection therapy or intraurethral suppository: These are both modalities where the medication is delivered directly to the tissues of the penis. Injection therapy has been around since the 1980s and is effective for producing erections but can cause prolonged erections or priapism events. Intraurethral suppositories use similar formulas to the intracavernosal injection but are rather a pellet that is inserted into the head of the penis. Both of these therapies can induce an erection in about 15 minutes but require in-office counseling and training to assure proper technique and dosage.

4. Penile implants: These are surgically implanted silicone tubes that offer a cure for erectile dysfunction. There are malleable implants made of semi-rigid rods that can be bent up for sexual function and down when not in use. Inflatable prostheses have expanding silicone cylinders in the cavernosa that attach to a pump hidden in the scrotum. The most common inflatable prosthesis also has a reservoir containing saline hidden deep in the pelvis. When the man wants to have sexual activity he compresses the pump in the scrotum that cycles saline from the reservoir and into the cylinders to give the man a rigid erection. After sexual activity, a button on the pump is compressed to allow the water to cycle back to the reservoir.

CASE 10.1

Mr. Reed is a 70-year-old retired engineer who presents with fatigue and "marriage problems" that have gradually gotten worse over the past decade. His appointment was made by his wife, who was worried that he has "not been himself" lately. He does not have a regular PCP but has a cardiologist due to a history of MI and stent placement shortly after his retirement at age 65. He reports skipping his past two cardiology appointments and discontinuing Lipitor due to muscle aches. He reports that he has recovered well from his heart attack and now works part-time in a motorcycle shop doing repairs. He has a long history of tobacco use and has quit several times in the past but has recently started again, although he endorses only smoking three to five cigarettes per day. He is interested in testosterone replacement therapy to "help him in the bedroom."

Upon further investigation, the patient endorses erectile dysfunction that started gradually about 10 years ago. His erectile function is about the same with masturbation as it is when attempting sex with his wife. He reports increased difficulty in achieving an erection and states that he can only get it "to half-mast." Further, he reports needing greater stimulation to maintain an erection. He denies morning erections and endorses decreased libido. He took some Viagra a few months ago that was given to him by a co-worker and it helped some. He states that his low libido has made erections worse. He takes a daily 81 mg aspirin and Clopidogrel 75 mg daily along with metoprolol 25 mg daily as prescribed by his cardiologist. He had a prescription for sublingual nitroglycerin shortly after his heart attack but no longer carries it and never used it in the past. His past medical history is significant for inguinal hernia repair in high school and possible TIA at the Newark airport 18 months ago.

Interprofessional Box

Direct-to-consumer advertising has increased the number of male patients asking for testosterone for help with sexual issues. Although Mr. Reed may have low testosterone, his ED is more likely vasculogenic due to arterial insufficiency. The history of smoking, MI, and TIA all point to vascular disease and the inability to achieve erection indicates possible arterial insufficiency. Since this patient does not have a PCP, it is important to connect him with primary care and have him follow up with cardiology. Princeton III criteria would likely place this patient in a low-risk category and indicate it is safe to resume sexual activity (Nehra et al., 2012), but the patient will need blood pressure monitored, possible medication changes (beta-blocker may contribute to ED), and counseling to quit smoking. Further, the patient may need a stress test to measure cardiac function prior to treatment for ED (Nehra et al., 2012).

It is important that patients seeking care for sexual dysfunction meet with a psychiatric provider, as the pathophysiology of sexual dysfunction can have a significant psychogenic component. A diminished arousal phase of the sexual response cycle can hamper a man's interest in sex and contribute to diminished libido (Burnett et al., 2018). Further, a feedback mechanism starting with decreased sexual performance and increased performance anxiety can contribute to a downward spiral in sexual function (Nimbi et al., 2020). The American Urological Association recommends referral to a mental health professional to "[i]ntegrate treatments into a sexual relationship" (Burnett et al., 2018). Thus, a patient may present to a psychiatric provider with an incomplete understanding of the comorbid conditions that contribute to sexual dysfunction in the aging male. Comanagement of the patient with sexual dysfunction is often key to successful treatment.

Evidence-Based Practice Box

Erectile dysfunction has a significant impact on mental and sexual health in the aging male (Korfage et al., 2009). Yet, erectile dysfunction is unidentified or undertreated in many older men (Dean, 2005). There is a high correlation between depression, aging, and erectile function (Seidman, 2002). It is therefore likely that a mental health provider will come into contact with older male patients who are suffering from sexual dysfunction. It is important to identify sexual dysfunction in the aging male, understand the iatrogenic contributions, and have an awareness of treatment options available (Perelman, 2011).

The American Urological Association recommends that patients with erectile dysfunction meet with mental health providers and be counselled on improvements in overall health (Gareri et al., 2014). Furthermore, men who have erectile dysfunction should be counseled on treatment options available (Burnett et al., 2018).

■ SEXUAL DYSFUNCTION IN THE AGED FEMALE

Sexual health can be broadly defined (according to the WHO, 2020) as encompassing one's behaviors, fantasies, and outcomes related to sexual health. Sexual health can be interpreted holistically encompassing one's "sexual gender, role, sexual orientation, eroticism, pleasure, intimacy and reproduction" (WHO, 2020). Female sexual dysfunction (FSD) is broadly defined and may encompass many psychological and somatic etiologies. A woman's sexuality can be altered by one's "interaction of biological, psychological, social, economic, political, cultural, legal, historical, religious and spiritual factors" (WHO, 2020). Consequently, FSD is more complicated and less understood than male sexual dysfunction due to gaps in research and women's' perceptions about sex when compared to males (Allahdadi et al., 2009). The prevalence of FSD among all women is between 38% and 63%, with even higher rates among older and postmenopausal women (ages 65–79 years) ranging from 68% to 86.5% (Addis, et al., 2006). Common symptoms of FSD include vaginal dryness, pain and discomfort with intercourse, diminished sense of arousal, and anorgasmia (Allahdadi et al., 2009).

FSD can negatively impact a woman's psychological and physiological wellness. In addition to psychological factors such as depression, trauma, past sexual abuse, and interpersonal factors there are many common organic disorders associated with aging that may be related to FSD (Ambler et al., 2012; Dahlen, 2019). Additionally, medication side effects may contribute to FSD. Therefore, a comprehensive health history and physical examination is important to consider and rule out all underlying causes which may be contributing to FSD.

The *Diagnostic and Statistical Manual of Mental Disorders Fifth Edition* (*DSM-5*) classifies FSD into three different diagnostic categories: female sexual interest/arousal disorder (FSIAD), genito-pelvic pain/penetration disorder (GPPD), and orgasmic disorder (American Psychiatric Association, 2013).

■ HORMONAL CHANGES

Estrogen is known to play a vital role in female sexuality and failure to maintain premenopausal estrogen levels may impact the physiological structures of the female genitourinary (GU) system (Ambler et al., 2012). One major function of estrogen is to provide pelvic muscle tone, elasticity, and genital tissue maintenance. When estrogen is not produced at optimal levels thinning of the vaginal mucosa may occur, resulting in dryness. "In menopausal women, the vaginal mucosa becomes attenuated, loses its rugae, and appears pale and almost transparent because of decreased vascularity" (Ambler et al., 2012). This is termed atrophic vaginitis. Additionally, chronically depleted estrogen causes the labia to become less sensitive to tactile stimulation. This loss of sensation results in less engorgement and swelling, and consequently, the labia are less likely to separate in response to sexual stimulation, ultimately leading to dyspareunia (Hofland & Powers, 1996). Other structures of the female GU system, such as the bladder, may also be affected. As a result of lower estrogen levels, the bladder may become thin, atrophic, and friable, which can be an organic cause of urinary incontinence, urinary frequency, dysuria, and cystitis after intercourse (Hofland & Powers, 1996). Additionally, low levels of free and total testosterone, androstenedione, and dehydroepiandrosterone sulfate have been shown to be a causative factor for low sexual desire in women (Panzer & Gray, 2009)

■ NEUROLOGIC DISORDERS

According to the National Multiple Sclerosis Society, multiple sclerosis is an autoimmune condition relating to damage to the myelin sheath in the central nervous system. The disruption of the nerve transmissions leads to an interference between brain, spinal cord, and body. Symptoms vary among individuals. The diagnosis of multiple sclerosis is dependent upon damage to two separate areas at different times within the CNS. Disease progression may alter one's sexual health as seen in delayed or difficulty achieving orgasms, altered genital sensation, or anorgasmia. Brainstem lesions disrupting the autonomic pathways and visual association have been associated with orgasmic dysfunction. (Winder et al., 2015). Commonalities seen in multiple sclerosis such as weakness, spasticity, impaired coordination, and slurred speech may inhibit one's desire for sexual intimacy. Medications commonly prescribed for MS, such as tricyclic antidepressants, and selective serotonin uptake inhibitors can result in decreased libido (Winder et al., 2015).

■ METABOLIC DISORDERS

According to Zamponi et al. (2020), correlations have been found between FSD and diabetes mellitus, dyslipidemia, and metabolic syndrome, and obesity with FSD was higher in women than in healthy controls. The study sample included 33 women with Type 1 diabetes and 39 healthy women, reflecting a small sample size. Researchers acknowledged sexual responses as being multicausal, with satisfaction in one's partner's sexual performance as playing a role in FSD; however, the potential prevalence of FSD in the study was attributed to neuropathy, angiopathy, and insulin administration. Limited data revealed the need for further research in the specialty.

According to Esposito et al. (2010), a study of 595 diabetic women aged 35 to 70 self-reported on a questionnaire on sexual dysfunctions. The mean age was 57.9 (± 6.9 years). Duration of diabetic onset reported at a mean of 5.2 years (± 1.5 years) and a mean A1C (HbA1C) level of 8.3 (± 1.3%) The Female Sexual Function Index had a cutoff point of 23. Prevalence of FSD among diabetic women was 53.4%, with diabetic menopausal women showing a prevalence of FSD at 64%. This was in strong comparison to non-menopausal women at 41% ($p < 0.001$). Age, metabolic syndrome, and atherogenic dyslipidemia were significantly associated with FSD. The meta-analysis showed diabetes could impact sexual function, especially when other comorbidities are present, and ultimately impact quality of life.

■ MEDICATIONS

A variety of different drug classes used in the aged female may be linked to FSD, including but not limited to antidepressants, antiepileptics, benzodiazepines, breast cancer treatment medications, antihypertensives (particularly beta-blockers), and opioids (Dahlen, 2019). Psychotropics are known to cause sexual dysfunction in most patients. According to Montejo et al. (2019), SALSEX study (n-2144) reported the frequency of antidepressant-induced sexual dysfunction for the total sample by sex and age. Over 80% of participants >50 years old (*n*-670) reported with overall sexual dysfunction while over 69% of participants >50 years old (*n*-670) reported with moderate to severe sexual dysfunction. Moderate to severe sexual dysfunction was categorized as decreased libido, delayed orgasms, anorgasmia, and lubrication dysfunction. Pharmacological classes included *selective serotonin reuptake inhibitors, serotonin-norepinephrine reuptake inhibitors, non-serotonergic antidepressants,* and *tricyclic antidepressants.* A research study by Jesus et al. (2018) evaluated relationships between antipsychotic drugs and sexual dysfunction. Alterations in menstrual cycles and prolactin levels when consuming first- and second-generation antipsychotic drugs were associated with decreased libido in female participants.

Assessment

In women reporting FSD, a complete history and physical examination should be completed with directed open-ended questions regarding sexuality and sexual health. In addition to a through health history, an emphasis should be placed on relationship status, sexual practices, past sexual abuse, and past sexual traumas. The use of evidence-based tools such as the Short Personal Experiences Questionnaire (SPEQ) or the Female Sexual Distress Scale (FSDS) may be employed when formulating a diagnosis.

■ FEMALE SEXUAL INTEREST/AROUSAL DISORDER

When healthcare providers diagnose female sexual interest/arousal disorder, they must consider if symptoms have persisted over 6 months and whether the disorder causes clinical distress in the individual. Also, they must take into consideration if there are outliers such as non-sexual mental disorders, severe relationship distress, or other significant stressors such as the effects of a substance or medication or other medical condition. When assessing the client, the healthcare provider will determine if there is a lack of or reduced sexual interest or arousal in at least three of the main diagnostic criteria. Criteria consist of an absence of reduced interest in sexual activities, erotic thoughts, or fantasies. The client may be unreceptive to a partner's initiation or sexual cues. The client may not have any sexual pleasure with reduced genital or non-genital sensations during most (75%–100%) sexual encounters

Assessment includes five factors related to etiology:

1. Partner factors, such as partner's health and sexual status

2. Relationship factors, including poor sexual desire and communication

3. Individual vulnerability, including one's self-esteem and body image

4. Cultural and religious factors related to one's inhibitions

5. Medical factors related to one's health status

Genito-Pelvic Pain/Penetration Disorder

Genito-pelvic pain penetration disorder is defined as having "vaginal pain during penetration during intercourse or marked vulvovaginal or pelvic pain during vaginal intercourse or penetration attempts."

Assessment includes five factors related to etiology:

1. Partner factors, such as partner's health and sexual status

2. Relationship factors, including poor sexual desire and communication

3. Individual vulnerability, including one's self-esteem and body image

4. Cultural and religious factors related to one's inhibitions

5. Medical factors related to one's health status

Sexual pain disorders such as dyspareunia describes recurrent or persistent genital pain. It occurs during sexual intercourse. Lack of lubrication is not the key factor, but it trends towards difficulties in interpersonal relationships. Vaginismus refers to spasms in the vaginal muscles during sexual intercourse. The involuntary spasms can occur continuously, preventing penetration. Vaginismus is related to distress or difficulties in interpersonal relationships. Comorbidities may include non-sexual mental disorders such as depression. The genito-pelvic pain disorder may also simultaneously impact one's sexual interest, arousal, and potential for orgasms.

Orgasmic Disorder

The female orgasmic disorder criteria are diagnosed when a person experiences no orgasmic sensations or delayed orgasmic sensations in 75% to 100% of all occasions. Symptoms are considered clinically significant and have persisted for over 6 months. The cause must not be related to severe relationship distress or other significant stressors, such as the effects of a substance or medication or other medical condition. Healthcare communication may be limited due to the client's willingness to discuss sexual health. Reported female orgasmic disorders have a range of variability from 10% to 42%. Orgasmic disorders are related to a multifactorial range of etiologies. (*DSM-5* TR). Sexual dysfunctions (2013).

Assessment includes five factors related to etiology:

1. Partner factors, such as partner's health and sexual status
2. Relationship factors, including poor sexual desire and communication
3. Individual vulnerability, including one's self-esteem and body image
4. Cultural and religious factors related to one's inhibitions
5. Medical factors related to one's health status

Treatment

The American College of Gynecology (2019) provides guidance to providers on the treatment of FSD using the best possible evidence available outlined by levels of evidence.

1. The following recommendations are based on good and consistent scientific evidence (Level A):

    ❏ Low-dose vaginal estrogen therapy is the preferred hormonal treatment for female sexual dysfunction that is due to genitourinary syndrome of menopause.

    ❏ Low-dose systemic hormone therapy, with estrogen alone or in combination with progestin, can be recommended as an alternative to low-dose vaginal estrogen in women experiencing dyspareunia related to genitourinary syndrome of menopause as well as vasomotor symptoms.

    ❏ Ospemifene can be recommended as an alternative to vaginal estrogen for the management of dyspareunia caused by genitourinary syndrome of menopause.

    ❏ Systemic DHEA is not effective and therefore is not recommended for use in the treatment of women with sexual interest/arousal disorders.

2. The following recommendations are based on limited or inconsistent scientific evidence (Level B):

    ❏ Psychologic interventions, including sexual skills training, cognitive–behavioral therapy (with or without pharmacotherapy), mindfulness-based therapy, and couples' therapy, are recommended as part of female sexual dysfunction treatment.

    ❏ A physical examination should be performed to diagnose female sexual dysfunction related to genitourinary syndrome of menopause before starting vaginal or systemic hormone therapy.

    ❏ Short-term use of transdermal testosterone can be considered as a treatment option for postmenopausal women with sexual interest and arousal disorders who have been appropriately counseled about the potential risks and unknown long-term effects.

❑ Evidence is insufficient to recommend for or against testosterone for the treatment of sexual interest and arousal disorders in premenopausal women. Sildenafil should not be used for the treatment of female interest/arousal disorders outside of clinical trials.

❑ Intravaginal prasterone, low-dose vaginal estrogen, and ospemifene can be used in postmenopausal women for the treatment of moderate-to-severe dyspareunia that is due to genitourinary syndrome of menopause.

❑ Estrogen or SERM therapy is not recommended for the treatment of female sexual dysfunction that is not due to a hypoestrogenic state.

❑ Vaginal carbon dioxide (CO_2) fractional laser for treatment of dyspareunia that is due to genitourinary syndrome of menopause should not be used outside of a research setting.

❑ Flibanserin can be considered as a treatment option for hypoactive sexual desire disorder in premenopausal women without depression who are appropriately counseled about the risks of alcohol use during treatment.

3. The following recommendations are based primarily on consensus and expert opinion (Level C):

❑ Obstetrician–gynecologists should initiate a clinical discussion of sexual function during routine care visits to identify issues that may require further exploration and to help destigmatize discussion of sexual function for patients.

❑ The initial evaluation of a patient with female sexual dysfunction symptoms may require an extended visit and should include a comprehensive history and physical examination to evaluate possible gynecologic etiologies.

❑ Laboratory testing typically is not necessary in the initial evaluation of female sexual dysfunction unless an undiagnosed medical etiology is suspected.

❑ If transdermal testosterone therapy is used in post-menopausal women with sexual interest and arousal disorders, a 3- to 6-month trial is recommended with assessment of testosterone levels at baseline and after 3 to 6 weeks of initial use to ensure levels remain within the normal range for reproductive-aged women. Transdermal testosterone therapy should be discontinued at 6 months in patients who do not show a response. If ongoing therapy is used, follow-up clinical evaluation and testosterone measurement every 6 months are recommended to assess for androgen excess. The long-term safety and efficacy of transdermal testosterone have not been studied.

❑ Pelvic floor physical therapy is recommended for the treatment of genito-pelvic pain and penetration disorders to restore muscle function and decrease pain.

❑ Lubricants, topical anesthesia, and moisturizers may help reduce or alleviate dyspareunia.

CASE 10.2

Mrs. Smith is a 62-year-old female who reports to the outpatient clinic with a chief complaint of painful urination that has become progressively worse over the last few months. She reports being married to the same partner for 41 years and reports they've had a very active sex life during their entire marriage, but it has slowed down over the last 10 years. The couple has four adult children, all of whom she carried to term with normal vaginal deliveries. Her associated symptoms include pain when "starting sex" and pain throughout the duration of the sexual encounter. This occurs every time she and her husband try to have sex. She states she has tried over-the-counter lubricants, but nothing really helps with the "dryness." She reports the inability to have an orgasm, stating she feels like she may "pee herself" during sex and has extremely painful urination for days after. She reports her last OBGYN appointment was

(continued)

greater than 10 years, stating, "I do not need to see an OBGYN if I don't have a period."

During your interview, you find that she takes metoprolol tartrate 50 mg twice daily for high blood pressure and fluoxetine 20 mg for "the worries." Sometimes, she takes an aspirin for "good measure." She states she is in "great health other than her blood pressure." She recently had cataract surgery but denies any other significant past medical or surgical history. She has never smoked and does not drink alcohol.

Interprofessional Box

Comorbid physical and psychiatric conditions may be present, which could contribute to FSD. Using interprofessional practice to engage other specialties such as specialist physicians, counselors, dieticians, wellness coaches, and other mental health practitioners may augment traditional treatment options for FSD.

Evidence-Based Practice Box

According to the American College of Obstetricians and Gynecologists (ACOG, 2019), a comprehensive sexual history should consider symptoms related to self-care, medication, partner or relationship factors, sexual function problems, physical activity, past injuries, sleep quality, body changes, and self-esteem. According to the American College of Obstetricians and Gynecologists (2019), sexual function has a relationship with medication administration. Its initiation and changes in dosage strength, whether increased or decreased can have a clinical impact on the client.

CRITICAL THINKING QUESTIONS

1. In older patients presenting with complaints of sexual dysfunction, what other etiologies and comorbidities are important to consider in the initial workup?

2. In older males with erectile dysfunction, why is co-management with primary care and other medical specialties necessary to properly address this disorder?

3. In older females, what evidence-based tools should be incorporated into your assessment of female sexual dysfunction and why?

4. What role do hormones play in female sexual dysfunction?

5. Which medical specialties would you anticipate including in your treatment plan?

REFERENCES

Male Section

Aversa, A., Bruzziches, R., Francomano, D., Natali, M., Gareri, P., & Spera, G. (2010). Endothelial dysfunction and erectile dysfunction in the aging man. *International Journal of Urology, 17*(1), 38–47. https://doi.org/10.1111/j .1442-2042.2009.02426.x

Biebel, M. G., Burnett, A. L., & Sadeghi-Nejad, H. (2016). Male sexual function and smoking. *Sexual Medicine Reviews, 4*(4), 366–375. https://doi.org/10.1016/j.sxmr.2016.05.001

Burnett, A. L., Nehra, A., Breau, R. H., Culkin, D. J., Faraday, M. M., Hakim, L. S., Heidelbaugh, J., Khera, M., McVary, K. T., Miner, M. M., Nelson, C. J., Sadeghi-Nejad, H., Seftel, A. D., & Shindel, A. W. (2018). Erectile dysfunction: AUA guideline. *The Journal of Urology, 200*(3), 633–641. https:// doi.org/10.1016/j.juro.2018.05.004

Carson, C. C., Kirby R. S., & Goldstein I. (1999). *Textbook of erectile dysfunction.* 1st ed. Isis Medical Media Ltd.

Dean, J. (2005). Characterisation, prevalence, and consultation rates of erectile dysfunction. *Clinical Cornerstone, 7*(1), 5–11. https://doi.org/10.1016/S1098-3597(05)80043-2

Dean, R. C., & Lue, T. F. (2005). Physiology of penile erection and pathophysiology of erectile dysfunction. *Urologic Clinics of North America, 32*(4), 379–395, v. https://doi.org/10.1016/j.ucl.2005.08.007

Francis, M. E., Kusek, J. W., Nyberg, L. M., & Eggers, P. W. (2007). The contribution of common medical conditions and drug exposures to erectile dysfunction in adult males. *The Journal of Urology, 178*(2), 591–596; discussion 596. https://doi.org/10.1016/j.juro.2007.03.127

Gareri, P., Castagna, A., Francomano, D., Cerminara, G., & De Fazio, P. (2014). Erectile dysfunction in the elderly: an old widespread issue with novel treatment perspectives. *International Journal of Endocrinology, 2014,* 878670. https://doi.org/10.1155/2014/878670

Hwang, T. I., Chen, H. E., Tsai, T. F., & Lin, Y. C. (2006). Combined use of androgen and sildenafil for hypogonadal patients unresponsive to sildenafil alone. *International Journal of Impotence Research, 18*(4), 400–404. https://doi.org/10.1038/sj.ijir.3901446

Korfage, I. J., Pluijm, S., Roobol, M., Dohle, G. R., Schröder, F. H., & Essink-Bot, M. L. (2009). Erectile dysfunction and mental health in a general population of older men. *The Journal of Sexual Medicine, 6*(2), 505–512. https://doi.org/10.1111/j.1743-6109.2008.01111.x

Liang, C. S., Ho, P. S., Chiang, K. T., & Su, H. C. (2012). 5-HT2A receptor-1438 G/A polymorphism and serotonergic antidepressant-induced sexual dysfunction in male patients with major depressive disorder: A prospective exploratory study. *The Journal of Sexual Medicine, 9*(8), 2009–2016. https://doi.org/10.1111/j.1743-6109.2012.02769.x

Maher, R. L., Hanlon, J., & Hajjar, E. R. (2014). Clinical consequences of polypharmacy in elderly. *Expert Opinion on Drug Safety, 13*(1), 57–65. https://doi.org/10.1517/14740338.2013.827660

Morton, L. (2017). Sexuality in the older adult. *Primary Care*, *44*(3), 429–438. https://doi.org/10.1016/j.pop.2017.04.004

Nehra, A., Alterowitz, R., Culkin, D. J., Faraday, M. M., Hakim, L. S., Heidelbaugh, J. J., Khera, M., Kirkby, E., McVary, K. T., Miner, M. M., Nelson, C. J., Sadeghi-Nejad, H., Seftel, A. D., Shindel, A. W., Burnett, A. L., & American Urological Association Education and Research, Inc. (2015). Peyronie's disease: AUA guideline. *Journal of Urology*, *194*(3), 745–753. https://doi.org/10.1016/j.juro.2015.05.098

Nehra, A., Jackson, G., Miner, M., Billups, K. L., Burnett, A. L., Buvat, J., Carson, C. C., Cunningham, G. R., Ganz, P., Goldstein, I., Guay, A. T., Hackett, G., Kloner, R. A., Kostis, J., Montorsi, P., Ramsey, M., Rosen, R., Sadovsky, R., Seftel, A. D., . . . Wu, F. C. W. (2012). The Princeton III Consensus recommendations for the management of erectile dysfunction and cardiovascular disease. *Mayo Clin Proceedings*, *87*(8), 766–778. https://doi.org/10.1016/j.mayocp.2012.06.015

Nimbi, F. M., Tripodi, F., Rossi, R., Navarro-Cremades, F., & Simonelli, C. (2020). Male sexual desire: An overview of biological, psychological, sexual, relational, and cultural factors influencing desire. *Sexual Medicine Reviews*, *8*(1), 59–91. https://doi.org/10.1016/j.sxmr.2018.12.002

O'Donnell, A. B., Araujo, A. B., & McKinlay, J. B. (2004). The health of normally aging men: The Massachusetts Male Aging Study (1987–2004). *Experimental Gerontology*, *39*(7), 975–984. https://doi.org/10.1016/j.exger.2004.03.023

O'Donnell, A. B., Travison, T. G., Harris, S. S., Tenover, J. L., & McKinlay, J. B. (2006). Testosterone, dehydroepiandrosterone, and physical performance in older men: results from the Massachusetts Male Aging Study. The *Journal of Clinical Endocrinology and Metabolism*, *91*(2), 425–431. https://doi.org/10.1210/jc.2005-1227

Perelman, M. A. (2011). Erectile dysfunction and depression: screening and treatment. *The Urologic Clinics of North*

America. *38*(2), 125–139. https://doi.org/10.1016/ j.ucl.2011.03.004

Sangkum, P., Levy, J., Yafi, F. A., & Hellstrom, W. J. (2015). Erectile dysfunction in urethral stricture and pelvic fracture urethral injury patients: diagnosis, treatment, and outcomes. *Andrology*, *3*(3), 443–449. https://doi. org/10.1111/andr.12015

Schulster, M. L., Liang, S. E., & Najari, B. B. (2017). Metabolic syndrome and sexual dysfunction. *Current Opinion in Urology*, *27*(5), 435–440. https://doi.org/10.1097/ MOU.0000000000000426

Seidman, S. N. (2002). Exploring the relationship between depression and erectile dysfunction in aging men. The *Journal of Clinical Psychiatry*, *63*(Suppl 5), 5–12; discussion 23–25.

Serefoglu, E. C., Smith, T. M., Kaufman, G. J., Liu, G., Yafi, F. A., & Hellstrom, W. J. G. (2017). Factors associated with erectile dysfunction and the Peyronie's disease questionnaire in patients with Peyronie disease. *Urology*, *107*, 155–160. https://doi.org/10.1016/j.urology.2017.05.029

Yafi, F. A., Jenkins, L., Albersen, M., Corona, G., Isidori, A. M., Goldfarb, S., Maggi, M., Nelson, C. J., Parish, S., Salonia, A., Tan, R., Mulhall, J. P., & Hellstrom, W. J. G. Erectile dysfunction. *Nature Reviews: Disease Primers.* 2016;2, 16003. https://doi.org/10.1038/nrdp.2016.3

Female Section

Addis, I. B., Van Den Eeden, S. K., Wassel-Fyr, C. L., Vittinghoff, E., Brown, J. S., Thom, D. H., & Reproductive Risk Factors for Incontinence Study at Kaiser Study Group. (2006). Sexual activity and function in middle-aged and older women. *Obstetrics and Gynecology*, *107*(4), 755–764. https://doi.org/10.1097/01.AOG.0000202398.27428.e2

Allahdadi, K. J., Tostes, R. C., & Webb, R. C. (2009). Female sexual dysfunction: Therapeutic options and experimental challenges. *Cardiovascular & Hematological*

Agents in Medicinal Chemistry, 7(4), 260–269. https://doi.org/10.2174/187152509789541882

Ambler, D. R., Bieber, E. J., & Diamond, M. P. (2012). Sexual function in elderly women: A review of current literature. *Reviews in Obstetrics & Gynecology, 5*(1), 16–27.

American College of Gynecology (ACOG) (2019). Female sexual dysfunction: ACOG practice bulletin summary, number 213. (2019). *Obstetrics and Gynecology, 134*(1), 203–205. https://doi.org/10.1097/AOG.0000000000003325

American Psychiatric Association. (2013). *Diagnostic and statistical manual of mental disorders.* 5th ed. American Psychological Association.

Dahlen, H. (2019). Female sexual dysfunction: Assessment and treatment. *Urologic Nursing, 39*(1), 39–46. https://doi.org/10.7257/1053-816X.2019.39.1.39

Esposito, K., Malorino, M. I., Bellastella, G., Giugliano, F., Romano, M., & Gugliano, D. (2010). Determinants of female sexual dysfunction in type 2 diabetes. *International Journal of Impotence Research, 22*(1), 79–84. https://doi.org/1038/lijir.2010.6

Hofland, S. L., & Powers, J. (1996). Sexual dysfunction in the menopausal woman: Hormonal causes and management issues. *Geriatric Nursing, 17*(4), 161–165. https://doi.org/10.1016/S0197-4572(96)80064-4

Female sexual dysfunction: ACOG practice bulletin summary, number 213. (2019). *Obstetrics and Gynecology, 134*(1), 203–205. https://doi.org/10.1097/AOG.0000000000003325

Jesus, R. A., Zardeto-Sabec, G., Quemel, F. S., & Santos, A. F. (2018). Relation between antipsychotic medicines and sexual dysfunctions. *Brazilian Journal of Surgery and Clinical Research, 22*(3), 31–36. https://www.mastereditora.com.br/periodico/20180504_105447.pdf

Montejo, A. L., Calama, J., Rico-Villademoros, R., Montejo, L., Carcia-Conzalez, N., Perez, J., & SALSEX Working Study Group. (2019). A real-world study on antidepressant-associated sexual dysfunction in 2144 outpatients: The

SALSEX I study. *Archives of Sexual Behavior, 48*, 923–933. https://doi.org/10.1007/s10508-018-1365-6

Panzer, C. & Gray, A. (2009). Testosterone replacement therapy in naturally and surgically menopausal women. *The Journal of Sexual Medicine, 6*(1), 8–18. https://doi.org/10.1111/j.1743-6109.2008.01128.x

Winder, K.., Seifert, F., Koehn, J., & Deutsch, M. (2015). Site and size of multiple sclerosis lesions enhanced or decreased female orgasmic disfunction. *Journal of Neurology, 262*(12), 2731–2738. https://doi.org/10.1007/s00415-015-7907-0

World Health Organization. (2020). *Defining sexual health.* https://www.who.int/reproductivehealth/topics/sexual_health/sh_definitions/en/

Zamponi, V., Mazzilli, R., Bitterman, O., Olana, S., Iorio, C., Festa, C., Giuliani, C., Mazzili, R., & Napoli, A. (2020). Association between type 1 diabetes and female sexual dysfunction. *BMC Women's Health, 20*(73), 1–7. https://doi.org/10.1186/s12905-020-00939-1

CHAPTER 11

MEDICATION ISSUES AND PRESCRIBING IN GEROPSYCHIATRY

MARIE SMITH-EAST
DAVID J. MOKLER

LEARNING OBJECTIVES

After reviewing this chapter, practitioners will be able to:

- recognize methods to assess medication issues when prescribing for the older adult
- identify contributing factors to medication issues
- summarize common black box warning(s) of medications for elderly patients
- initiate ways to decrease medication issues and prescribing in the older adult

■ INTRODUCTION

Geriatric psychiatric care in today's world requires comprehensive and astute participation among healthcare providers as older adults are living longer—some with complex, co-occurring chronic medical conditions (Birch, 2016). The emphasis in healthcare is on outcomes and quality care. Advanced practice nurses have the distinguishing ability to provide care that incorporates undergraduate nursing experiences, advanced education in pharmacology, and pathophysiology. The purpose of this chapter is to highlight medication issues and to offer guidance for prescribing for geriatric populations across healthcare settings. Advanced practice nurses must have a clear understanding of their role, methods for assessing issues, and an evaluation of needs to provide high-quality care.

■ A REVIEW OF MEDICATION ISSUES AND THE PRACTITIONER'S ROLE

Although the overall healthcare team in a variety of settings (home health, hospitals, clinics, or nursing rehabilitation facilities) should be well aware of the treatment plan for an older adult (65 and older), it is the practitioner's role to be prudent about medications prescribed. The practitioner should consider multiple facets related to the older adult's care when prescribing medication.

First, there must be a thorough review of the patient's history to prevent harm to the individual and essentially to all. This is often referred to as due diligence (Fishalow, 1975). Understandably, the patient's history may come from a variety of sources, particularly if the patient does not recall all of their past medications or even their current medications. The practitioner should contact (which can easily be done via phone) family members, guardians, or close friends (with consent) who could provide a description or account of the patient's history with medications. Close attention to a history of side effects, adverse effects, and doses should be completed. Some hospital facilities allow for team members to contact pharmacies to find the last time a medication was filled and by whom.

Ensuring that past hospital, clinic, or nursing rehabilitation records have been attained for a psychiatric review of records is important. This triangulation of collecting a patient's medication history can assist the advanced practice nurse with providing care that is tailored to the patient and prevent unnecessary medication trials or ineffective treatment. Furthermore, the practitioner can also use their thorough review of the patient's history in discussing a treatment plan and providing education with family members who have power of attorney (common in geriatric populations) and may be reluctant to start medications due to troublesome outcomes from past experiences.

■ ADHERENCE DOSING AND DISPENSED MEDICATION

Medication management for elderly patients with any chronic medical illness in itself can be challenging (Yap et al., 2016). Depending on the area in which the patient is being treated regularly, taking into consideration the ability of the older adult to manage their medications will assist with proper adherence. The timing and cost of psychiatric medications for an individual who may be on a fixed income should assist the prescriber with creating a treatment plan that is individualized. For example, tricyclic antidepressants have been found to contribute to orthostatic hypotension, particularly in the elderly (Darowski et al., 2009). Less commonly, selective serotonin reuptake inhibitors (SSRI) could also contribute to orthostatic hypotension; thus, dosing such medications once a day at bedtime may be a strategy that could help to reduce any occurrences related to falls. If the patient does not have a daily pill container or cannot remember to take a medication during a particular time of the day, once-daily dosing is another strategy that could be used.

■ METHODS TO ASSESS MEDICATION ISSUES

Medication issues may not always appear glaringly evident in terms of missed doses. Asking the patient what their daily routine is with regard to their medications or simply what medications are they currently taking could provide insight into any issues related to medications. Asking questions specifically related to the time of day the patient is actually taking the medications prescribed could foster useful information that the practitioner can use to provide appropriate care.

■ MEDICATION RECONCILIATION

The Joint Commission (2016) emphasizes that as part of quality care, safety nets such as medication reconciliation should be considered during the transition of care for managing medications. Most facilities have a protocol that includes medication reconciliation by nursing staff that is recommended on admission, discharge, every care transition and transfer, and at every provider appointment. In the event that medication reconciliation information is not easily accessible, this step should not be skipped. Despite the treatment setting, medication reconciliation each time the patient meets with the provider should be completed. Patients may have a change of medical medications, which could affect interactions or effectiveness of prescribed psychiatric medications.

■ PHARMACY FLAGS

Often integrated in the electronic health record or pharmacy records is a pharmacy alert that provides a description of interactions of medications prescribed. Understanding the mechanism of action regarding certain psychiatric medications and how they can be induced or inhibited by other medications is integral. In the event that the electronic health record or pharmacy does not have the information readily available, there are other methods that can be used, such as drug interaction tools or pharmaceutical books (such as *Stahl's Essential Psychopharmacology*) that provide information on medications that may work best. Although not a requirement, collaboration with the pharmacist regarding medications of which the prescriber may be unsure can be helpful.

For example, in certain facilities, there may be a flag regarding the use of benztropine for extrapyramidal symptoms due to potential for adverse effects in the elderly, and an alternative such as amantadine may be warranted. Some pharmacy flags may occur where the practitioner is notified that the patient is on more than one antidepressant. Close attention and justification should be provided regarding antidepressants that are in different classes, such as SSRIs (e.g., sertraline) versus serotonin-norepinephrine reuptake inhibitors (SNRIs; e.g., venlafaxine), and the risk for serotonin syndrome. Documentation regarding provided education to the patient and an awareness of the different classes of medications should be noted.

■ ANTI-CHOLINERGIC SYNDROME AND SEROTONIN SYNDROME

Professionals should be aware of two syndromes that may cause significant complications in patients who take multiple medications: anticholinergic syndrome and serotonin syndrome.

Many classes of drugs commonly prescribed or bought over-the-counter have a mechanism of action that involves actions to block acetylcholine receptors. These receptors are involved in cognitive function in the brain and in many actions involving the parasympathetic nervous system. Classes of drugs that have these actions include anti-depressants, neuroleptic medications, GI medications, allergy medications, insomnia medications, and cold medications. These drugs can cause many effects, including urinary retention, constipation, tachycardia, and blurred vision. Importantly, these drugs may also cause confusion, decreased cognitive function, and memory loss. In older patients, these changes in CNS function may be mistaken for worsening of dementia. All drugs that have anticholinergic properties should be avoided in the elderly.

Similarly, many drugs may increase levels of serotonin in the central nervous system. These include anti-depressants, trazodone, and opioids. Symptoms may be minor or may involve major symptoms such as coma and death.

■ DRUG INTERACTION TOOLS

Credible and updated drug interaction tools are beneficial when prescribing psychiatric medications for patients who are taking multiple medical medications. While there are some applications that may be available on devices such as smartphones or tablets, oversight regarding the credibility of the drug interaction tool in addition to comparing the tool's results with others is needed. Various pharmacies, organizations, and electronic health records systems such as Cerner are sources for online "drug interaction checker" (Drugs.com, 2018) tools. After deciding which medications to prescribe, it is good practice to review for any interactions. Some electronic prescribing programs are automatically integrated into the electronic prescribing platform before a script is sent to the pharmacy providing any warnings. After reviewing any medication interactions, adjustments such as lower dosing, tapering one medication for another, cross-titration, providing education, and documenting education provided to the patient is warranted.

■ POSSIBLE CAUSES OF MEDICATION ISSUES AND PRESCRIBING

There may be instances where medication is not warranted. Therefore, assessing the needs of the geriatric patient will assist with alternative methods of treatment. For example, a patient who frequently requests to go home or to call a family member multiple times within an hour in a residential setting after just conversing with the family member may have other needs that nursing staff could fulfill. Staff should be trained on how to meet the needs of patients through thorough assessment and offering a variety of resources. Family members can be asked about activities that the patient enjoys. Offering to connect patients to individual therapy, group therapy, one-on-one activities, or other resources available in the community can be beneficial and vary depending on the treatment setting.

Another common issue that is reported in geriatric care settings is a high turnover rate among staff which can lead to issues that affect patient care (Blomberg et al., 2013). Meetings with administration and brief in-services with nursing staff that are reflective of and include their beliefs about providing geriatric care can address some of the issues that can affect overall care. An interdisciplinary team approach (even by phone) that incorporates how each area can maximize the effectiveness of care can provide additional insights, such as physical therapy or psychotherapy scheduling times that are best suited for the individual patient, as some medications could have side effects affecting these activities.

■ PHYSICAL ISSUES

Some psychotropic medications have side effects that can exacerbate the physical symptoms of the elderly client. Therefore, it is important to assess the timing and dosing of newly administered medications. For example, if a patient has a medical medication that contributes to nighttime awakening to use the bathroom, the prescriber must be cognizant of any medications given at night that could contribute to falls. Alternative timing for medications, such as evening versus bedtime, are considerations that can be implemented. As part of the assessment for neuroleptic medications, an Abnormal Involuntary Movement Scale must be initiated after treatment once every 6 months and every 3 months for patients older than 50 years of age (Psych Congress, 2017). Involuntary movements should be screened at baseline in order to not be confused with any other medical condition (such as Parkinson's disease) for which a referral to a neurology specialist should be made.

■ GERIATRIC DOSING AND MEDICATIONS TO AVOID

Imperative to care for older adults is the need to consider geriatric dosing and the close monitoring of labs. For example, in a patient with an estimated glomerular filtration rate (eGFR) of less than 60, indicating severe renal impairment, makers of the medication

Namenda XR instruct that the prescriber should not exceed 14 mg per day (Allergan, 2016). The key to geriatric dosing, aside from being aware of the patient's current labs, is that often a particular medication may not be contraindicated in the geriatric population, just recommended to be given at a lower dose or with the appropriate *Diagnostic and Statistical Manual of Mental Disorders, Fifth Edition (DSM-5)* diagnosis.

There are also some valuable drugs that should not be used or used with caution in the older patient, as well as drugs that are safe to use. The Beers Criteria are classes of drugs that should be avoided in the older patient (American Geriatrics Society Beers Criteria Update Expert Panel, 2015). These lists were last updated in 2015. In addition, O'Mahony et al. (2014) developed a screening tool for older people's prescriptions (STOPP) and a screening tool to ensure right treatment (START). These references are additional tools for determining appropriate medications in older patients.

■ MULTIPLE PRESCRIBERS

Patients who have been prescribed psychotropic medications should have continuity of care with the same psychiatric provider. If not, patients could have a surplus of medications, which could put them at risk there is a history of overdose. Furthermore, coordination of care must be completed if there are concerns that certain medications prescribed by another provider could interfere with the effectiveness of treatment. Respectfully, an acknowledgment and documentation regarding any discussions that involve concerns regarding potential issues with medications with multiple prescribers must be completed.

■ RISKS VERSUS BENEFITS

Risks versus benefits are terms commonly utilized in mental health to address the use of psychotropic medications. Outlined risks and benefits conducive to the patient's current status should be considered and re-evaluated at continuous intervals. Although additional research is necessary to quantify a risk-to-benefit ratio, the benefits of the use of psychotropic medications should certainly outweigh the risks.

■ BLACK BOX WARNINGS

The United States Food and Drug Administration (FDA) has provided specific black box warnings for patients on medications such as Haldol (Thom et al., 2017), Celexa (FDA, 2012), Trazodone (FDA, 2014), and Geodon (FDA, 2005a) that have QT/QTc prolongation established as greater than 450 ms (FDA, 2005b). A QT/QTc prolongation greater than 500 ms is a cause for discontinuation as this could lead to arrhythmias, which would result in death (FDA, 2005b). A baseline EKG should be ordered on any patient starting on such medications and completed again during their course of treatment.

For elderly patients with dementia-related psychosis, a black box warning of increased mortality is associated with the use of all antipsychotic medications (Yan, 2008). Again, outlining the risks versus benefits and the appropriateness of the medication given the patient's diagnosis is necessary when considering the use of antipsychotic medications in the elderly. Extensive education should be provided to the patient and caregiver. For olanzapine injection, there is a black boxed warning for post-injection delirium/sedation syndrome. Thus, it is only available at a registered healthcare facility and not given directly to a patient (CMS, 2015).

■ DIAGNOSING AND ACCOMPANYING PRESCRIPTION

Currently, the Centers for Medicare and Medicaid Services (2016) described the quality measure of the use of antipsychotics in older patients in the inpatient hospital setting for inappropriate use to exclude the following diagnoses: schizophrenia, Huntington's disease, bipolar disorder, and Tourette's syndrome. While the quality measure may exclude certain patients that have such diagnoses, it is important to ensure that the relevant diagnosis accompanies the patient's prescription. The appropriateness of a continued prescription should be re-evaluated on a regular basis and include assessing for the minimum effective dose necessary—particularly for individuals with co-occurring dementia diagnoses.

■ GRADUAL DOSE REDUCTION

Many nursing home rehabilitation facilities have a gradual dose reduction (GDR) program, which may consist of monthly meetings with the psychiatric prescriber, social worker, director of nursing, pharmacist, and medical director. The purpose of the meeting is to review the patient's diagnosis, symptoms, and need for medication. A GDR is implemented for patients on any psychotropic medications to gradually reduce to the minimum effective dosage.

■ INTERDISCIPLINARY MEETINGS

Interdisciplinary meetings are warranted in each setting where a patient may be receiving multiple services. For example, a meeting with the physical therapy team, occupational therapy team, and recreational team may provide additional insights on the timing of medications and improvement in symptoms. There could be areas of concern in which a one-to-one meeting (even by phone) could be completed to discuss concerns or how to improve individualized care.

■ CONCLUSION

Medication issues and prescribing in geriatric psychiatric care can involve multiple factors that must be considered and addressed in order to encourage safe, quality, and effective care. The advanced practice nurse must be able to recognize and address medication issues that can occur when prescribing psychotropic medications, particularly in the geriatric population where there is high vulnerability and complexity. The use of interdisciplinary collaboration can be beneficial to the advanced practice nurse providing care in various settings where the needs of the geriatric patients can change.

CASE 11.1 **THE MAN CLINICIANS HAVE BEEN AFRAID TO PROVIDE TREATMENT TO**

A 75-year-old African American male presents with a history of severe depression and a new onset of agitated behaviors. The staff at his assisted living facility report staff have been afraid to provide care as he will hit or kick the person providing care. He has medical diagnoses of Parkinson's disease, type I diabetes, chronic kidney disease, and hypertension. You look over his medication list and notice that the patient is also on a stimulant. His family reports he has been on it for years and insists he should have it increased for attention deficit disorder.

1. How would you approach treatment for this patient?

2. How could you implement an interdisciplinary approach to include the family members with regard to the treatment plan?

3. What labs and medications would you order (if warranted)?

Interprofessional Box

After evaluating the 75-year-old male, he informs you that he is having a difficult time keeping track of all of the medications that he is taking and when. He reports that his daughter, who typically helps him with his medications, has been

(continued)

working extra hours and has not had the time to help him as much, and he "does not want to bug her with my problems."
Consider:

Medication reconciliation of all medications from all providers from whom patient currently receives medications

Collaborating with primary care physician for a reduction in polypharmacy

Use of a medication box/dispenser

Obtaining consent to discuss additional assistance or solutions with family/caregiver

Referral for case management/social services for additional resources

Evidence-Based Practice Box

Increased complexities related to prescribing medication for the older adult population involve safety concerns associated with polypharmacy, adverse drug reactions, cognitive impairment, falls, and hospitalizations (Koronkowski et al., 2016). Kukreja et al. (2013) further explained that patients with a diagnosis of schizophrenia, schizotypal, and delusional disorders were more likely to have polypharmacy, while better neurocognitive functioning was associated with decreased chances of psychiatric medication polypharmacy. Advanced practice nurses can help to reduce issues related to prescribed medications in the older adult population through comprehensive assessment, management, and maximizing strategies that improve drug therapy while decreasing adverse drug reactions (Cope, 2013). A holistic approach that involves considerations for comorbidities and chronic illnesses in the older population can result in improved care.

REFERENCES

Heyman, D. L. (2008). *Control of communicable diseases manual* (19th ed.). American Public Health Association.

Allergan. (2016). *Namenda: Highlights of prescribing information.* https://www.allergan.com/assets/pdf/namendaxr _pi

American Geriatrics Society Beers Criteria Update Expert Panel. (2015). American Geriatrics Society 2015 Updated Beers Criteria for potentially inappropriate medication use in older adults. *Journal of the American Geriatrics Society, 63*(11), 2227–2246. https://doi.org/10.1111/jgs.13702

Birch, D. (2016). Comprehensive geriatric assessment of a patient with complex needs. *Nursing Older People, 28*(4), 16–20.

Blomberg, K., James, I., & Kihlgren, A. (2013). Meanings over time of working as a nurse in elderly care. *The Open Nursing Journal, 7,* 107–113. https://doi .org/10.2174/1874434620130726005

Centers for Medicare and Medicaid Services. (2013). Atypical antipsychotic medications: Use in adults. Retrieved from https://www.cms.gov/Medicare-Medicaid-Coordination/ Fraud-Prevention/Medicaid-Integrity-Education/ Pharmacy-Education-Materials/Downloads/atyp -antipsych-adult-factsheet11-14.pdf

Centers for Medicare and Medicaid Services. (2016). *Use of antipsychotics in older patients in the inpatient hospital setting (AP) measure.* https://www.cms.gov/Medicare/ Quality-Initiatives-Patient-Assessment-Instruments/ MMS/Downloads/Hospital-MDM_AP-Public-Comment -Summary-Report_FINAL.pdf

Cope, D. G. (2013). Polypharmacy in older adults: The role of the advanced practitioner in oncology. *Journal of the Advanced Practitioner in Oncology, 4*(2), 107. https://doi .org/10.6004/jadpro.2013.4.2.5

Darowski, A., Chambers, S. A. C., & Chambers, D. J. (2009). Antidepressants and falls in the elderly. *Drugs &*

Aging, 26(5), 381–394. https://doi.org/10.2165/00002512 -200926050-00002

Drugs.com. (2018). *Drug interactions checker.* https://www .drugs.com/drug_interactions.html

Fishalow, S. E. (1975). The tort liability of the psychiatrist. *The Bulletin of the American Academy of Psychiatry and the Law, 3*(4), 191–230.

The Joint Commission. (2016). *Transitions of care: Managing medications.* https://www.jointcommission.org/ assets/1/23/Quick_Safety_Issue_26_Aug_2016.pdf

Koronkowski, M., Eisenhower, C., & Marcum, Z. (2016). An update on geriatric medication safety and challenges specific to the care of older adults. *The Annals of Long-Term Care, 24*(3), 37.

Kukreja, S., Kalra, G., Shah, N., & Shrivastava, A. (2013). Polypharmacy in psychiatry: A review. *Mens Sana Monographs, 11*(1), 82. https://doi.org/10.4103/0973-1229.104497

O'Mahony, D., O'Sullivan, D., Byrne, S., O'Connor, M. N., Ryan, C., & Gallagher, P. (2014). STOPP/START criteria for potentially inappropriate prescribing in older people: Version 2. *Age and Ageing, 44*(2), 213–218. https://doi .org/10.1093/ageing/afu145

Psych Congress. (2017). *Trivia: How often should you screen for tardive dyskinesia?* https://www.psychcongress.com/ article/trivia-how-often-should-you-screen-tardive -dyskinesia?page=2

Thom, R. P., Mock, C. K., & Teslyar, P. (2017). Delirium in hospitalized patients: Risks and benefits of antipsychotics. *Cleveland Clinic Journal of Medicine, 84*(8), 616–622.

U.S. Food and Drug Administration. (2005a). *Geodon.* https://www.accessdata.fda.gov/drugsatfda_docs/ label/2005/020825s015,017,020919s005,006lbl.pdf

U.S. Food and Drug Administration. (2005b). *Guidance for the industry.* https://www.fda.gov/downloads/drugs/ guidancecomplianceregulatoryinformation/guidances/ ucm073153.pdf

U.S. Food and Drug Administration. (2012). *FDA drug safety communication: Revised recommendations for Celexa (citalopram hydrobromide) related to a potential risk of abnormal heart rhythms with high doses.* https://www.fda .gov/drugs/drugsafety/ucm297391.htm

U.S. Food and Drug Administration. (2014). *Medication guide: Tradozone hydrochloride.* https://www.accessdata .fda.gov/drugsatfda_docs/label/2015/071196s062lbl.pdf

Yan, J. (2008). *FDA extends black-box warning to all antipsychotics.* https://psychnews.psychiatryonline.org/doi/ 10.1176/pn.43.14.0001

Yap, A. F., Thirumoorthy, T., & Kwan, Y. H. (2016). Medication adherence in the elderly. *Journal of Clinical Gerontology and Geriatrics*, *7*(2), 64–67. https://doi.org/10.1016/j .jcgg.2015.05.001

CHAPTER 12

ELDER ABUSE

MARIE SMITH-EAST

LEARNING OBJECTIVES

After reviewing this chapter, practitioners will be able to:

- recognize signs and symptoms of elder abuse
- summarize laws pertinent to elder abuse
- describe factors that contribute to elder abuse
- identify how to respond to needs related to elder abuse

■ INTRODUCTION

According to the National Institute on Aging (2019), hundreds of thousands of adults over the age of 60 are abused each year. Elder abuse is often under the umbrella of elder mistreatment, which includes abuse, neglect, and exploitation of individuals aged 65 or older (National Research Council, 2003). The purpose of this chapter is to describe risk factors, types of elder abuse, and approaches for prevention and treatment. Advanced practice nurses must be prepared to report as mandated by law and be advocates for prevention and treatment while meeting the needs of elderly patients to ensure quality care.

■ THE PRACTITIONER'S ROLE

There are many settings in which the advanced practice nurse could encounter elder abuse, such as nursing homes, assisted living, and even the homes of the patient or family member where the patient currently resides. Therefore, the advanced practice nurse must be vigilant through providing a thorough assessment and deciding the necessary treatment plan (including reporting if warranted), as each state varies with mandatory reporting laws for healthcare professionals. Elder abuse is a crime and there are statutes that exist to protect older adults, with the extent of such punishments varying state by state (U.S. Department of Justice, 2020). The role of the advanced practice nurse is to advocate for prevention and know when and how to report abuse while protecting the rights of older adults, as elder abuse can lead to life-threatening physical injuries and chronic psychological outcomes (WHO, 2018).

■ RISK FACTORS

Elder abuse is defined as an act or lack of an appropriate action that results in harm or distress to an older person aged 60 years or older (WHO, 2018). Risk factors associated with the vulnerability to abuse in the older adult can involve individual, relational, community, and societal characteristics (Centers for Disease Control and Prevention, 2018). Many of the risk factors are described as a level of need, such as being socially isolated and having a mental impairment (National Council on Aging, 2019a). Poor physical and mental health also contributes to susceptibility to abuse in the older adult (WHO, 2018).

> **Individual.** Elderly women are at a higher risk of neglect and financial abuse when they are widowed, particularly in cultures where the women have an inferior social status (WHO, 2018). Having poor mental and physical health can contribute to elder abuse as there could be instances of an expectation of trust in assisting with ailments that could be violated. Older adults with higher rates of major depressive disorder and post-traumatic stress disorder have been identified as most impacted by mistreatment (Acierno et al., 2017). Older adults with disabilities, dementia, or Alzheimer's disease are more likely to experience abuse or neglect (National Council on Aging, 2019a).

Relationships. Poor family relationships and shared living spaces can be a risk factor for elder abuse (WHO, 2018). In the instance of the abuser or perpetrator, a dependency on the elderly person's financial backing can increase the risk of abuse. Not having enough time to manage caring for the older adult can also increase the risk of elder abuse (WHO, 2018).

Community. Lack of social support can contribute to elder abuse (WHO, 2018). Social isolation of caregivers and older adults are risk factors for elder abuse (Acierno et al., 2017; National Council on Aging, 2019a; WHO, 2018).

Society. A society that perpetuates stereotypes of older adults as weak or dependent, systems of inheritance that affect the distribution of resources within families, long-term care facilities with poor physical environment or poorly trained staff, and lack of funds to assist with paying for care all contribute to risk factors for elder abuse (WHO, 2018).

■ TYPES OF ELDER ABUSE

There are many warning signs and symptoms of elder abuse that can be recognized in both the victim (the older adult) and the perpetrator (the abuser). Some signs and symptoms of abuse can be more obvious than others. However, in all instances, suspected abuse should be addressed.

■ PHYSICAL ABUSE

Physical abuse is the use of physical force that may result in bodily harm to an individual, such as hitting, biting, cutting, pushing, burning, kicking, pinching, or slapping. Common signs and symptoms of physical abuse include bruises, broken bones, abrasions, and burns (National Center on Elder Abuse, 2019). The less obvious signs and symptoms can include the older adult's sudden change in behavior, the caregiver's refusal to allow visitors to see the person alone, and laboratory findings of overdose or underdose of prescribed medications (National Center on Elder Abuse, 2019). The advanced practice nurse should look at any findings of abuse collectively; for example, if a patient recently had a fall, the injuries should be consistent with a fall (e.g., if the patient fell on their left leg and there is a noticeable bruise on their left leg) and fall precautions should be in place. An older adult's report of being physically abused should be assessed for immediate danger and steps to protect the patient from any future occurrences must be addressed. Specific steps for reporting immediate danger and suspected abuse are discussed further in this chapter.

■ EMOTIONAL OR PSYCHOLOGICAL ABUSE

Emotional or psychological abuse involves verbal or nonverbal acts that cause distress such as verbal assaults, yelling, threats, humiliation, and harassment (National Center on Elder Abuse, 2019; National Institute on Aging, 2019). The less obvious signs and symptoms of emotional or psychological abuse can include the older adult being extremely withdrawn or non-communicative or the caregiver socially isolating the patient from others or regular activities (National Center on Elder Abuse, 2019). In nursing homes or assisted living facilities, verbal or emotional mistreatment, especially to individuals with dementia, may be downplayed as the patient possibly not remembering the interaction, yet these behaviors still should not occur and should be addressed. Furthermore, in being vigilant, the advanced practice nurse should make comparisons to baseline behavior and whether reported behaviors are new onset and different from previously assessed visits.

■ SEXUAL ABUSE

Sexual abuse involves sexual contact of any type that is not consensual with an elderly person, particularly with those who are unable to provide consent, and can include sexually explicit photographing and sexual assault or battery (National Center on Elder Abuse, 2019). Signs and symptoms of sexual abuse include bruises around genital areas and torn or stained clothing. Less obvious signs and symptoms of sexual abuse include unexplained genital or sexually transmitted infections (National Center on Elder Abuse, 2019). Testing an elderly patient for a sexually transmitted infection is not routinely done without cause, and any findings that result in a positive result should be considered collectively as part of the assessment. Each facility in which the advanced practice nurse is employed may have different procedures to follow with regard to reporting. Nevertheless, elder abuse should be reported to authorities (immediately to the police for immediate danger) and suspected abuse should be reported via the Elder Abuse Hotline at 1-800-677-1116. There is also an Elder Abuse Locator, which is a public service of the United States Administration on Aging, that is provided for anyone who suspects abuse: https://eldercare.acl.gov/Public/Index.aspx

■ FINANCIAL ABUSE

Financial abuse involves illegal or inappropriate use of an elderly patient's money, property, or assets (National Center on Elder Abuse, 2019). Signs and symptoms of financial abuse include unauthorized or unexplained transfer or withdrawal of an elderly person's funds, disappearance of valuable possessions, unpaid bills despite the availability of funds, abrupt changes to financial documents or a will, and forged signatures on the elderly person's titled possessions (National Council on Aging, 2019a). An elderly patient may report financial abuse to the advanced practice nurse, who should assess further, listen, provide empathy, and address concerns accordingly with treatment team members (and if necessary report).

■ NEGLECT

Neglect involves failure to provide responsibilities to an elder such as pay for care, or to provide necessary care that is essential for life such as food, water, shelter, and safety (National Center on Elder Abuse, 2019). Signs and symptoms of neglect include malnutrition or dehydration, unsanitary living conditions, untreated health issues, untreated bed sores or pressure marks (which could also be related to physical abuse), and unsafe living conditions. Neglect can occur not only in the elderly's home, but also in assisted living facilities and nursing homes.

■ ABANDONMENT

Abandonment includes deserting an elderly person whom the caregiver had assumed responsibility of providing care for (National Center on Elder Abuse, 2019). A sign of abandonment other than the elderly person explicitly reporting abandonment can include leaving an elderly person at a public location or facility. The prudent advanced practice nurse should further assess any reports or signs of abandonment and address any concerns. For example, a patient may disclose to the advanced practice nurse that their caregiver has left them multiple times at home for days at a time without food. This should be distinguished from self-neglect. For instance, the advanced practice nurse may inquire about neglect of the elderly person to the caregiver and the caregiver may report that the patient has been refusing to eat. Elder self-neglect involves the failure of the elderly person to provide themselves with care with regard to food, hygiene, medication, living environment, and safety precautions (Dong, 2017). The complexity of the level of elder abuse can vary in instances where the elderly person lives alone versus with a caregiver. Regardless of the setting, the key components that must be assessed for is adequate water, clothing, hygiene, living environment, and safety.

■ HEALTHCARE FRAUD

In July 2017, 412 individuals were arrested by U.S. federal investigators in healthcare fraud schemes targeting the elderly (AARP, 2018). Healthcare fraud is not limited to caregivers and can be committed by healthcare staff, including clinicians and other healthcare workers (National Institute on Aging, 2019). Examples of healthcare fraud include falsifying health insurance claims, billing for care that was not provided, or overcharging services (National Institute on Aging, 2019). Advanced practice nurses should be aware of this type of fraud and should avoid signing blank insurance claim forms and authorization to bill for services not provided, and maintain accurate records of healthcare services provided to avoid civil and license penalties that could result in criminal liabilities.

■ PREVENTION

There are many programs in place to assist with preventing elder abuse and assisting older adults in exercising their rights in acting against abuse (National Center on Elder Abuse, 2019). Advanced practice nurses can assist caregivers at the start of providing treatment in connecting them to resources that provide respite care, stress management, and training on dementia (WHO, 2018). In many nursing home and assisted living facilities, case managers who are on the interdisciplinary treatment team can assist with referrals. For victims of elder abuse, research has demonstrated that the degree of social support an older adult perceives in their life is a protective factor against the consequences of elder abuse (Acierno et al., 2017). Screening, spreading awareness, and collaborating with interdisciplinary sectors to encourage additional support can prove beneficial.

■ CAREGIVER STRESS

According to the National Council on Aging (2019a), almost 60% of cases of elder abuse and neglect involve a family member as the perpetrator, with two thirds being the elderly person's adult children or spouses. Continual assessment that involves providing any additional support for the caregiver as needed should be integrated into the advanced practice nurse's holistic assessment of the care provided to the elderly patient. Offering caregiver support services can be beneficial as caregiver support even after abuse has occurred can reduce the likelihood of reoccurrence (WHO, 2018).

■ REPORTING

Although there are estimates that are as high as 5 million older adults suffering from abuse each year, it is estimated that only one in 14 cases of abuse are reported to authorities (National Council on Aging, 2019a). Laws in most states require healthcare professionals to report suspected abuse or neglect. The National Council on Aging (2019b) provides an elder locator regarding state reporting laws and other resources; however, if the situation is life-threatening, the local police must be called for immediate help. When making the call, the name of the individual suspected of being abused or neglected, address, and contact information will be needed as well as information about why you are concerned (some states do not require that you identify yourself when making the report and the agency receiving the report are prohibited from disclosing you as a reporter to the suspected victim or abuser; National Center on Elder Abuse, 2019).

■ TREATMENT

Providing support for older adults who have experienced abuse is necessary as part of their recovery. Associated trauma that resulted in subsequent mood disorders from emotional, physical, and sexual abuse should be treated as such which can include medication management and individual therapy. For example, medication management would follow the diagnosis for the mood disorder and additional resources depending on the setting and needs of the patient should be addressed. In a nursing home setting, an interdisciplinary approach that involves slowly integrating the patient into the social environment, one-on-one support, and medication management addressing symptoms related to anxiety, depression, and/or nightmares would be treated based on the standards that already exist for such conditions (such as medications that are SSRIs, Buspirone, or Prazosin). Individualized treatment plans should address how to connect patients to any necessary resources such as transportation, legal support (as there are national networks that can provide free legal representation for patients), and financial assistance (Administration for Community Living, 2017), which again are provided through the Eldercare Locator resource and hotline provided.

Considerations for the effects of the dynamics related to repercussions for the caregiver should also be addressed within the interdisciplinary approach to treatment as there may be instances where the abused individual feels a sense of guilt, shame, and/or denial for disclosing the abuse. Rodogno (2008) explained that restorative practices can be used an an intervention to maintain the relationship among family members and the patient if a family member may have been the one inflicting the abuse on the elderly patient since the abuse can affect the overall family dynamics. Restorative practices can involve therapy that process the emotions that are experienced as a result of the abuse. The interdisciplinary approach to treatment can encourage engagement of emotions such as guilt, shame, empathy, and hope in addition to feelings of anger, humiliation, fear, and disgust (Rodogno, 2008).

■ CONCLUSION

Elder abuse is a crime and as members of the healthcare team, advanced practice nurses are mandated to report immediate and suspected abuse. There are various forms of elder abuse that should be identified, assessed further, and include a treatment plan. Each setting may vary in available interdisciplinary systems responding to the needs of the elderly person abused, yet the overall goals for treatment outcomes remain the same—to improve and protect the lives of the elderly.

CASE 12.1 THE ELDERLY PATIENT WITH DEMENTIA SUSPECTED OF BEING NEGLECTED

A 70-year-old Caucasian male presents with a history of early stage dementia and cardiovascular disease. He recently had a stroke and is unable to care for himself; thus, his adult son and daughter-in-law moved in with him to help. He is expected to start physical therapy in the home next week. During your home visit, you notice his room smells like urine, food stains are all over his clothes, and there are sores on the heels of his feet. The patient appears unexplainably withdrawn and discusses he's hungry as his son and daughter-in-law have been too busy to get him anything to eat and he's not sure where all his money has gone. You are worried that his family is neglecting and possibly financially abusing him.

1. What would you consider addressing first in your assessment?

2. How would you address concerns with the patient and the caregiver?

3. How could you implement an interdisciplinary approach to include other members of the treatment team regarding concerns you have for the patient?

Interprofessional Box

After evaluating a 70-year-old male, he mentions to you he is afraid to tell you what is really going on [regarding questions you have asked regarding elder abuse] at home as he does not want to "lose everything," including "the only person I have left" (his caregiver).

Consider:

Using nonjudgmental language, including asking questions addressing safety and what the patient would like to do in addition to educating the patient on what can be done

(*continued*)

Reporting any cases of suspected mistreatment (a requirement based on the state you live or under the Elder Justice Act)

Relaying your concerns to local adult protective services or calling the Eldercare Locator help line

Developing interventions designed to empower clinicians in preventing, identifying, and reporting signs of elder abuse, and after reporting, encourage interdisciplinary restorative practices

Utilizing agencies in the community for additional resources and support

Evidence-Based Practice Box

Advocates of evidence-based practice emphasize that a "one-size-fits-all" approach is not always suitable in developing implementation strategies that address a specific population or issue (National Center on Elder Abuse, 2011). Evidence-based programs targeting the prevention of elder abuse should make cultural considerations, hold perpetrators accountable, and provide support for elders that are affected. Improved health outcomes for the elderly or reduced elder abuse can occur when interdisciplinary approaches with evidence-based practice are used, which in turn can enhance sustained funding of such programs (National Center on Elder Abuse, 2011).

REFERENCES

American Association of Retired Persons. *Meet the faces of fraud.* https://www.aarp.org/money/scams-fraud/info-2017/elder-fraud-scam-stories.html

Acierno, R., Hernandez-Tejada, M. A., Anetzberger, G. J., Loew, D., & Muzzy, W. (2017). The National Elder Mistreatment Study: An 8-year longitudinal study of outcomes.

Journal of Elder Abuse & Neglect, 29(4), 254–269. https://doi.org/10.1080/08946566.2017.1365031

Administration for Community Living. (2017). *Protecting rights and preventing abuse.* https://acl.gov/programs/protecting-rights-and-preventing-abuse

Centers for Disease Control and Prevention. (2018). *Risk and protective factors.* https://www.cdc.gov/violenceprevention/elderabuse/riskprotectivefactors.html

Dong, X. (2017). Elder self-neglect: Research and practice. *Clinical Interventions in Aging, 12,* 949–959. https://doi.org/10.2147/CIA.S103359

National Center on Elder Abuse. (2011). *The use of evidence-based practice for elder abuse programs.* Retrieved from https://ncea.acl.gov/NCEA/media/Publication/The-Use-of-Evidence-Based-Practices-for-Elder-Abuse-Programs.pdf

National Center on Elder Abuse. (2019). *Elder rights resources.* https://ncea.acl.gov/Resources/Elder-Rights.aspx

National Council on Aging. (2019a). *Elder abuse facts.* https://www.ncoa.org/public-policy-action/elder-justice/elder-abuse-facts/

National Council on Aging. (2019b). *State resources.* https://ncea.acl.gov/Resources/State.aspx

National Institute on Aging. (2019). *Elder abuse.* https://www.nia.nih.gov/health/elder-abuse

National Research Council. (2003). *Elder mistreatment: Abuse, neglect, and exploitation in an aging America.* National Academies Press.

Rodogno, R. (2008). Shame and guilt in restorative justice. *Psychology, Public Policy and Law, 14*(2), 142–176. https://doi.org/10.1037/a0013474

U.S. Department of Justice. (2020). *Elder abuse and elder financial exploitation statutes.* https://www.justice.gov/elderjustice/prosecutors/statutes?field_statute_state=MD&field_statute_category=All

World Health Organization. (2018). *Elder abuse.* https://www.who.int/news-room/fact-sheets/detail/elder-abuse

CHAPTER 13

FAMILY DYNAMICS

MARIE SMITH-EAST

LEARNING OBJECTIVES

After reviewing this chapter, practitioners will be able to:

- identify personal, social, and cultural factors related to family dynamics that can have an impact on care
- describe the practitioner's role in addressing family dynamics during care
- summarize approaches to address issues related to family dynamics, including care for the caregiver, in practice

■ INTRODUCTION

Family dynamics for the elderly patient are essential for a better understanding of the many components that can impede or enhance care. As an advanced practice nurse, consideration for family dynamics adds to an overall holistic approach to treatment and is often what differentiates nursing care. First, assessing the level of independence or what has changed in the management of the older adult's day-to-day activities is vital. Older adults who were once the primary caregiver of the household but now depend on their adult child or children to manage their finances may have difficulty adjusting to the new roles. Second, family roles could interfere with the manner in which future affairs are handled, such as the plan of care differing from what a healthcare surrogate or medical power of attorney would want to see happen. Third, family dynamics could vary widely by culture, which could also impact the plan of care for the older adult. This chapter will highlight how different factors related to family dynamics could impact care and how advanced practice nurses could approach care in such instances.

■ THE PRACTITIONER'S ROLE

Depending on the setting in which the advanced practice nurse is employed, family dynamics can manifest in various ways. For example, an elderly patient living in an assisted living facility may express feelings of loneliness related to the lack of visits from their adult children. Another elderly patient may express vulnerability related to feeling like a burden to their adult children with whom they live in a private practice setting. Regardless of the manner in which family dynamics may be discussed, the advanced practice nurse must be diligent in assessment to provide an approach to treatment that encompasses contributing factors that can affect the patient's overall care. Therefore, the practitioner's role is to assess diligently, encourage clear communication among all involved, intervene with medications to stabilize mood if necessary, and refer to other members of the treatment team regarding additional resources, such as referrals for community resources, social services, and therapy where warranted..

■ INDEPENDENCE

Imagine a life where you drove yourself to work everyday or managed your own finances, yet due to circumstances beyond your control, you no longer have the ability to do such things for yourself anymore. Many elderly patients often describe losing their independence as one of the most difficult components to aging, attributed to a phenomenon described as a succession of losses that are gradual or sudden (Pitt, 1998). Advanced practice nurses must be aware that physical, psychological, and social losses could trigger symptoms of depression (Singh & Misra, 2009) and thus must be incorporated into the plan of care.

Resistance to care, often manifested as being angry for having to be cared for, feeling frightened or like a burden to others, and memory loss (such as not understanding why one must be cared for) are all considerations that must be assessed. While medications can be prescribed for symptoms associated with physical loss or to slow the process of memory loss, incorporating other resources into the plan of care that address each issue could provide more of an integrative approach leading to more comprehensive and sustained improvements.

Many older adults may also seek additional social support through church members, neighbors, or community organizations, while others may withdraw from social circles (Population Reference Bureau, 2009). Assessing what life may have been like for the older adult prior to any losses could help the treatment team and family members in targeting an approach that is individualized and more likely to be agreeable for the older adult. For example, involving social services to provide transportation to church once a week could provide a type of respite care for an adult child taking care of an elderly parent who has always enjoyed attending church services each week.

■ FAMILY ROLES

Family roles can change over time. For instance, elderly patients who may have become widowed or divorced or now have grandchildren present the potential for role conflicts in families where there is a shared role of responsibility for the elderly patient (Zelezna, 2018). Some adult children may have both elderly parents to care for, or adult siblings may disagree on how to manage care for their elderly parent, in some instances possibly regressing to earlier roles or conflicts. Assessing for overburden of responsibilities of the older adult and the adult child or children is necessary in order to distinguish how to approach care.

While symptom management related to decreasing any mood changes in the elderly patient may be necessary, the social context related to care must also be addressed. For example, if an elderly patient is now having to take care of grandchildren in exchange for staying at their adult child's home, the dynamics around this expectation should be explored and alternatives offered if these lead to negative outcomes.

Furthermore, Silverstein and Giarrusso (2010) discussed how parenting styles, busy schedules, and the spouses of the older adult's child or children could influence parental feelings of ambivalence towards the older adult for whom they now must provide care. Incorporating different perspectives related to family members and the older adult in relationship to overall care should be provided. Considerations for individual and family therapy could be offered to target the psychosocial components related to care.

■ CULTURE, BELIEFS, AND COMMUNITY

"Approximately 34 million Americans, more than 10% of the U.S. population, were estimated to have served as an unpaid caregiver for someone age 50 or older in the year 2015" (Kaplan & Berkman, 2016, p. 1). In some cultures, there may be an understanding that an elderly person is to be taken care of in the home(s) of their adult children. For example, in China, India, Bangladesh, and Singapore, there are family support laws (referred to as filial-support laws) that support the needs of the elderly within a family by requiring that it is "a statutory duty for adult children to financially support their parents who are unable to provide for themselves" (Serrano et al., 2017, p. 788). In addition, there are religious beliefs that individuals may have that view taking care of the elderly is an honor rather than a task. For example, religion has been found to contribute to positive aging (often referred to as a source of comfort, support, and hope) for elderly individuals (Malone & Dadswell, 2018) while also impressing upon an obligation that many adult children of the elderly have to take care of their parents who once took care of them. Although the underlying belief that elderly parents must be taken care of, the extent of this belief can vary depending on the patient's belief system. For example, various religions have beliefs that may be similiar or different on how care should be provided among family members in the older stages of life, particularly among Judaism (Edelstein et al., 2017; Jewish Values Online, 2020; Jotkowitz et al., 2005), Christianity (Collins & Hawkins, 2016), and Islamic religions (ICNA, 2016). Considerations for the patient's belief system must be made during assessment by the advanced practice nurse in order to enhance individualized care.

Elderly individuals in rural environments encounter increased barriers to access to healthcare, which can include having less access to long-term care support, compared to urban environments and therefore may rely often on family and friends in order to access resources as well as caregiving support (Bouldin et al., 2018). For example, in rural areas where transportation may be required in order to attend healthcare appointments or to get groceries, social connectedness within the community can also be of assistance with meeting such needs. Social connectedness is defined as a subjective evaluation that involves having meaningful relationships with other individuals or groups, including caring for others or feeling cared for and feeling part of a community (Bouldin et al., 2018).

Increased life expectancy has also led to multiple generations co-existing at the same time in the household, further adding to the complexity involved in providing care (Silverstein & Giarrusso, 2010). Assumptions should not be made regarding the older adult's cultural beliefs, and asking clarifying questions regarding the older adult and family members can include:

- How do you view how elders should be taken care of?
- In your family, how have elders typically been taken care of?
- Who typically takes the role of taking care of everyone in your family?
- What are your religious beliefs and how do they relate to the care of any elders in your family?

Answers to questions related to culture and beliefs can start the process of understanding how family dynamics contribute to an individual's overall mood. Listening and providing alternatives with input from the overall treatment team, in addition to symptom management with medications (if indicated), can assist in the approach of utilizing a better understanding of family dynamics as a solution rather than a problem. Depending on the answers, questions related to culture and beliefs, referrals regarding social services, or even respite care may be warranted. Advanced practice nurses can often start to see additional benefits to mood when social factors are addressed. Discussing arrangements and a schedule for care divided among family members may be favorable, particularly in families where the expectation is that family members work together to provide care.

■ CARE FOR THE CAREGIVER

After assessing the needs of the patients and overall family with regard to providing care for the elderly patient, it is important to also address the needs of the caregiver. Some government agencies as well as private community organizations, including churches within the community, can provide respite care. Resources available within the caregiver's community could include caregiving support groups, with many even being specific to the caregiver's needs such as Alzheimer's caregiver support and within different modalities such as in-person or even online (Family Caregiver Alliance, 2019). The advanced practice nurse can work with interdisciplinary teams to make referrals to such resources within the community.

■ CONCLUSION

In summary, understanding that the fundamentals of caregiving involves not only the person being cared for but also the person providing care is crucial to the core of family dynamics. Maintaining communication among all parties involved and balancing the needs of both the caregiver(s) and the older adult is crucial to successful care and managing family dynamics. Advanced practice nurses are positioned to provide holistic care that utilizes a holistic approach while considering the role of family dynamics in providing care.

| CASE 13.1 | THE ROLE OF FAMILY DYNAMICS IN PROVIDING CARE TO AN ELDERLY WOMAN |

A 75-year-old Hispanic female recently moved into her oldest daughter's home after her husband died a year ago. Her youngest daughter, who is present during the appointment, explains to you she notices every time she visits her mom now she seems to be crying and is refusing to eat. She doesn't think her mom likes her sister's new husband and is not sure if her sister has the time to take care of her mom plus her three adolescent nephews.

1. What questions would you consider asking the older adult first as part of your assessment?

2. How would you address concerns related to care among family members? How might culture play a role in the family dynamics?

3. How could you implement an interdisciplinary approach to include other members of the treatment team regarding concerns you have for the patient?

Interprofessional Box

After evaluating a 75-year-old female, she mentions to you that she does not feel there is any medication that will help with the stress of dealing with her family and tearfully explains that she often feels alone. She reports she is not suicidal but she does not believe things within her family dynamics will ever get better.

Consider:

Evaluating and addressing any views/concerns regarding starting individual and family therapy and referral for case management for additional activities that may be available in the community as social support, including group therapy

Making available resources or local agencies that provide in-home therapy and support (such as transportation, and/or meal services) if necessary

Evidence-Based Practice Box

As older adults are living longer, many families are often providing some degree of care and/or support to an elderly family member. Evidence-based practice interventions that support caregiving tasks are beneficial in several ways, including helping to improve skills/problem-solving abilities for those to whom they are providing care (Gitlin et al., 2005). Caregivers of elderly patients who are balancing caregiving with other responsibilities may feel an increased sense of burden (Yu et al., 2015), which can certainly affect family dynamics. Advanced practice nurses can help to improve outcomes between caregivers and their patients through understanding family roles and dynamics, and providing education as well as support during the healthcare process.

REFERENCES

Bouldin, E. D., Shaull, L., Andresen, E. M., Edwards, V. J., & McGuire, L. C. (2018). Financial and health barriers and caregiving-related difficulties among rural and urban caregivers. *The Journal of Rural Health*, *34*(3), 263–274. https://doi.org/10.1111/jrh.12273

Collins, W. L., & Hawkins, A. D. (2016). Supporting caregivers who care for African American elders: A pastoral perspective. *Social Work and Christianity*, *43*(4), 85–103.

Edelstein, O. E., Band-Winterstein, T., & Bachner, Y. G. (2017). The meaning of burden of care in a faith-based community: The case of ultra-Orthodox Jews (UOJ). *Aging & Mental Health*, *21*(8), 851–861. https://doi.org/10.1080/13607863.2016.1175418

Family Caregiver Alliance. (2019). *Support groups*. https://www.caregiver.org/support-groups

Gitlin, L. N., Hauck, W. W., Dennis, M. P., & Winter, L. (2005). Maintenance of effects of the home environmental skill-building program for family caregivers and individuals with Alzheimer's disease and related disorders. *The Journals of Gerontology Series A: Biological Sciences and Medical Sciences*, *60*(3), 368–374. https://doi.org/10.1093/gerona/60.3.368

Islamic Circle of North America. (2016). *Importance of parents: An Islamic perspective*. https://www.icna.org/importance-of-parents-an-islamic-perspective/

Jewish Values Online. (2020). *What is the Jewish view on obligation to care for aging parents?* http://www.jewishvaluesonline.org/36

Jotkowitz, A. B., Clarfield, A. M., & Glick, S. (2005). The care of patients with dementia: A modern Jewish ethical perspective. *Journal of the American Geriatrics Society*, *53*(5), 881–884. https://doi.org/10.1111/j.1532-5415.2005.53271.x

Kaplan, D. & Berkman, B. (2016). *Family caregiving for older people*. https://www.merckmanuals.com/home/older-people's-health-issues/social-issues-affecting-older-people/

family-caregiving-for-older-people?query=Family%20 Caregiving%20for%20the%20Elderly

Malone, J., & Dadswell, A. (2018). The role of religion, spirituality and/or belief in positive ageing for older adults. *Geriatrics*, *3*(2), 1–16. https://doi.org/10.3390/geriatrics3020028

Pitt, B. (1998). Loss in late life. *BMJ*, *316*(7142), 1452–1454. https://doi.org/10.1136/bmj.316.7142.1452

Population Reference Bureau. (2009). *Aging, family structure, and health*. https://www.prb.org/familyandhealth/

Serrano, R., Saltman, R., & Yeh, M. J. (2017). Laws on filial support in four Asian countries. *Bulletin of the World Health Organization*, *95*(11), 788–790. https://doi.org/10.2471/BLT.17.200428

Silverstein, M., & Giarrusso, R. (2010). Aging and family life: A decade review. *Journal of Marriage and Family*, *72*(5), 1039–1058. https://doi.org/10.1111/j.1741-3737.2010.00749.x

Singh, A., & Misra, N. (2009). Loneliness, depression and sociability in old age. *Industrial Psychiatry Journal*, *18*(1), 51. https://doi.org/10.4103/0972-6748.57861

Yu, H., Wang, X., He, R., Liang, R., & Zhou, L. (2015). Measuring the caregiver burden of caring for community-residing people with Alzheimer's disease. *PLoS One*, *10*(7), e0132168. https://doi.org/10.1371/journal.pone.0132168

Zelezna, L. (2018). Care-giving to grandchildren and elderly parents: Role conflict or family solidarity? *Ageing & Society*, *38*(5), 974–994. https://doi.org/10.1017/S0144686X16001434

CHAPTER 14

PALLIATIVE CARE AND END-OF-LIFE ISSUES

MARIE SMITH-EAST

LEARNING OBJECTIVES

After reviewing this chapter, practitioners will be able to:

- describe ethical considerations of providing geriatric palliative care
- explain differences between end-of-life care and palliative care
- identify symptoms management during end-of-life mental healthcare
- evaluate patient and family needs when providing end-of-life care
- summarize approaches to palliative care and billing/fraud issues in palliative care

■ INTRODUCTION

The end of life can have so many meanings for various cultures. Moments that lead to the end of life are of particular importance, as the longstanding effects and impressions on family and friends will continue after the patient's death. Considering all of the factors that can correspond with end-of-life care, advanced practice nurses should reflect on how to best help patients and their families during this crucial time. While describing end-of-life care, it is important to distinguish that end-of-life care is not synonymous with palliative care. End-of-life care (also referred to as hospice) involves allowing the individual to live a quality of life that expresses their wishes about where to receive care and to die with dignity. While both end-of-life care and palliative care can improve the quality of life in an individual with a terminal illness, palliative care is not just for individuals nearing the end of their lives since palliative care involves a relief of pain that provides the individual with a quality of life without suffering, which could describe individuals with severe illness who require pain and symptom management (American Psychological Association, 2019). Therefore, end-of-life care can include palliative care. Palliative care includes a multidisciplinary team approach to care for individuals with a serious illness (even if it is not a life-threatening illness) and encompasses any age or stage of the illness (American Psychological Association, 2019) while enriching the lives of patients and their families (World Health Organization, 2018). The purpose of this chapter is to describe the goals, management of symptoms, and needs while providing palliative and end-of-life care for the elderly within the realm of mental healthcare. For elderly patients who may have difficulty accessing care or require assistance due to the lack of decision-making capacity, such vital components must also be incorporated when addressing treatment options.

■ THE PRACTITIONER'S ROLE

The approach to geriatric palliative care is integrative and involves an interdisciplinary method of care with the goal of relieving pain and suffering to improve the quality of life for patients and their families (World Health Organization, 2011). Yet there are barriers to the use of palliative care by patients and families due to inaccuracies of knowledge and/or negative beliefs among the general public that palliative care is hospice and essentially "giving up" and succumbing to death (Taber et al., 2019). Thus, one of the roles of the advanced practice nurse is to provide education regarding the differences between end-of-life and palliative care, which can include further resources (such as referrals within the interdisciplinary team). Ganzini et al. (2003) further explained that providing mental healthcare alongside palliative care warrants further consideration, as there is often a balancing act that occurs between managing terminal illness with mental health in which symptoms may worsen. Therefore, the advanced practice nurse within the realm of mental healthcare involves assessment and respect for persons while utilizing approaches within the palliative care framework.

■ MODIFICATIONS IN LEVEL OF CARE

To start, when providing palliative care from the perspective of the mental health advanced practice nurse for elderly patients, the clinician must work collaboratively with the interdisciplinary team regarding current orders in place to keep the patient comfortable. Palliative care focuses on providing patients with relief from pain, stress, and symptoms related to serious illness (Fairman & Irwin, 2013). Thus, the advanced practice nurse must assess for patient and family goals for care that assists in managing symptoms and is consistent with supportive care. Some patients and families may ask that certain medications are withheld or lowered in the context of advanced planning while monitoring for the minimization of symptoms to prevent any harm or make any declining mental illness worse. The advanced practice nurse must document how any treatment including medications is contributing to the palliation of symptoms with the improvement of quality of life as a goal.

Another modification to care involves providing continuous one-to-one care or supervision, which may already be provided by some palliative care agencies. For example, some providers may elect for the patient to have one-to-one care by a home care assistant during end-of-life care if the patient is at risk for falls. In these instances, the advanced practice nurse may find it beneficial to have the home care assistant provide a log of the patient's behavior to include as part of the overall assessment when determining medications or any other factors that could contribute to the patient's overall well-being. Some nursing home facilities may not have the ability to provide a care assistant continuously on a one-to-one basis during this time; however, considerations for this type of care should be implemented.

■ ETHICAL CONSIDERATIONS AND HEALTH DISPARITIES

When discussing an approach to end-of-life care that involves possibly discontinuing any medications or encouraging medications that may assist with comfort, ethical considerations involving treatment is a must. During end-of-life, patients may have impaired communication skills or an inability to make informed decisions; thus, Martins Pereira et al. (2018) discussed the importance of preserving autonomy for end-of-life care decisions. To reduce paternalism during end-of-life care, advanced planning is encouraged. Advanced planning involves individuals creating medical advanced directives regarding what their wishes are in the event that they are unable to do so for themselves.

Within the realm of advanced planning, it is imperative to recognize that palliative care disparities exist as individuals with serious mental illness are less likely to access and receive palliative care (Cai et al., 2011; Chochinov et al., 2012). For example, nursing home residents with schizophrenia (compared to their matched cohort) were less likely to see specialists, less likely to be prescribed pain medications, and less likely to receive palliative care (Chochinov et al., 2012). As palliative care disparities among individuals with serious mental illness can be complex, there are multiple factors that could possibly contribute to such disparities. Further research is necessary to better understanding personal, social, and provider factors.

■ CAPACITY, COMPETENCY, AND DO-NOT-RESUSCITATE ORDERS

Based on the Nurse Practice Act for the state in which the advanced practice nurse lives, the laws that govern determination of capacity, or even the facility in which an elderly patient receives treatment, advanced practice nurses may or may not be allowed to sign off paperwork deeming a patient incapacitated or without ability to make informed decisions (such as with regard to their healthcare treatment). In such instances, the advanced practice nurse must work with the physician, who would evaluate for capacity. Another aspect of this subject to consider is competency, which is a judicial finding by the court where an advanced practice nurse or physician can suggest lack of capacity based on assessment findings but cannot determine competency (Sorrentino, 2014). Thus, the advanced practice nurse must be diligent in understanding the laws governing advanced practice according to the state in which they practice, as a state could be deemed as a reduced practice or restricted state for advanced practice nurses, yet have laws that allow nurse practitioners to determine capacity. For example, New York is categorized as a reduced practice state for advanced practice nurses (AANP, 2019) but allows determination of incapacity by a nurse practitioner or physician and the ability for nurse practitioners to write do-not-resuscitate (DNR) orders (MOLST, 2019).

■ PLAN OF CARE

Determining a plan of care for patients receiving palliative care must be interdisciplinary. With regard to medications, the patient should be evaluated for medications that may be necessary in order to continue to providing comfort measures, which will first require medication reconciliation of all medications. Medications should be assessed for appropriateness and overall target symptoms during this time of care. Masman et al. (2015) highlighted that of the common psychiatric medications used during palliative care, such as midazolam and haloperidol, there is little evidence that supports these drugs as licensed for this approach. Although psychiatric palliative care does not explicitly provide guidelines regarding addressing symptoms of palliative care already associated with medical conditions (Trachsel et al., 2016), evaluating the patient on a case-by-case basis for behaviors that may warrant medications must be consistent with the patient's advance planning and of the basis of palliative care. Higher considerations for medications that are most likely to result in less side effects or that will target a particular symptom is essential.

Symptom management. In deciding how to provide treatment during end-of-life care for a dying patient, the advanced practice nurse should do so collaboratively with collaborating clinicians, the patient, and caregivers and/or family. Autonomy must be given with considerations that the patient is able to process information and is free from being coerced (Bailyn & Rubin, 2003). During end-of-life care, it is possible that the patient may refuse to eat or is taking only minimal fluids, which can add to the complexity of medical versus psychiatric care. In such instances, it is critical to view the patient holistically and symptoms that are managed should include a combination of meeting patient needs as well as collaboration to address mood symptoms related to depression, anxiety, personality changes, and confusion (Bailyn & Rubin, 2003). While the exact timing related to the terminal illness can be difficult to predict and can add to anticipatory anxiety, working with the primary care clinician to promote treatment, referral for psychotherapy, and adjusting any current mood stabilizer or antipsychotic treatments appropriately while promoting an understanding of the patient's psychiatric needs during end-of-life care with family and caregivers can prove beneficial to the patient's overall quality of life during this time.

Patient and family needs. Caregivers, family, and friends should be provided with additional resources during end-of-life care to provide additional support. While patients may get better to a point where they are deemed acceptable to come off of hospice, advanced practice nurses must be mindful that the status of the patient could change at any time. The support provided to the patient also extends to that of the caregiver, family, and friends involved; for example, a husband who stays day and night by his wife's side and does not want to go home to get any rest could benefit from caregiver support through case management services. The role of the advanced practice nurse during this time also considers the patient's spiritual beliefs and culture while still remaining objective in the care that is provided.

■ BILLING ISSUES AND FRAUD

Unfortunately, there have been cases of Medicaid and Medicare fraud where patients during end-of-life care were fatally overmedicated for profit (Curtin, 2019). In 2017, Medicare fraud resulted in $60 billion dollars to United States taxpayers a year (Schulte, 2017). Thus, in providing palliative care that optimizes the quality of life for individuals with terminal illness, the advanced practice nurse must be attentive to the services and time billed while also considering legal and ethical issues related to treatment. Advocating and being aware of services provided to the patient during end-of-life care must be carefully considered to avoid issues that could lead to fraud, such as medications chosen and doses utilized. For example, Curtin (2019) highlighted a court case in which a nursing supervisor directed other nurses to overmedicate hospice patients, such as increasing Ativan and morphine, to speed up the process of death for profit. Medicare fraud reporting can be done by phone or email through a "tip" line and many places of employment will also protect the employee for any reporting. Regardless, clinicians must be aware of their time spent and billing to avoid any payment errors that could result in incorrect billing.

■ CONCLUSION

End-of-life care and palliative care are not synonymous and the approach for each type of care, particularly as it relates to mental healthcare, should be considered. The advance practice nurse must be cognizant of various issues that may arise when providing end-of-life care. An interdisciplinary approach to palliative care is not only beneficial, but necessary in order to achieve certain treatment goals. The multidisciplinary team approach when providing palliative care should include a treatment plan that is discussed by needs among the team, the patient, and their family.

CASE 14.1   THE ELDERLY PATIENT WITHOUT A LIVING WILL?

A living will has not been determined for an 85-year-old female. The patient expressed worry about her recent assessment by her primary care provider as there is fear that the patient might have a terminal illness and she is not sure what will happen to her pets if anything were to happen to her. She also explained that her adult children do not get along and she fears about any healthcare decisions that would be made if anything were to happen to her.

1. What questions would you consider asking the older adult first as part of your assessment?

2. How would you address her concerns related to care and family members?

3. How could you implement an interdisciplinary approach to include other members of the treatment team regarding concerns you have for the patient?

Interprofessional Box

After evaluating an 85-year-old female, her adult daughter, who is the patient's caregiver and is in the room when you are getting ready to leave, inquires about what will happen to her mother during the end-of-life care, such as if the patient will continue medications or therapy and if palliative care services are available.

Consider:

Collaborating with the attending medical clinician regarding medical medications that the patient will continue in addition to any other therapies

Collaborating with other clinicians that are also providing any therapies (such as physical, speech, or occupational therapy) regarding plan of care

Referral for case management services

Resources in the community regarding palliative care

Referral for caregiving support services

Providing education regarding your role in providing and approach to patient's end-of-life care

Evidence-Based Practice Box

In palliative psychiatric care, the first step is to communicate the current diagnosis, prognosis, symptoms, and then management (Trachsel et al., 2016). Reassessment during end-of-life care is necessary as the patient's symptoms can change during the course of treatment. Referrals for caregiver support and family needs should be made in addition to interdisciplinary communication. The goal of palliative care should continue with preserving dignity and encouraging

(*continued*)

autonomy and acceptance as much as possible during this time. The advanced practice nurse can have an impact not only in the patient's life, but also the caregiver's in assessing for appropriateness and benefits in the approach to care.

REFERENCES

American Association of Nurse Practitioners. (2019). *State practice environment.* https://www.aanp.org/advocacy/state/state-practice-environment

American Psychological Association. (2019). *Older adults and palliative end of life care.* https://www.apa.org/pi/aging/programs/eol/end-of-life-factsheet.pdf

Bailyn, R., & Rubin, J. (2003). *Psychiatric treatment challenges at the end of life.* https://www.aagponline.org/clientuploads/Clinical%20View/clinicalView_v2n1.pdf

Cai, X., Cram, P., & Li, Y. (2011). Origination of medical advance directives among nursing home residents with and without serious mental illness. *Psychiatric Services, 62*(1), 61–66. https://doi.org/10.1176/ps.62.1.pss6201_0061

Chochinov, H. M., Martens, P. J., Prior, H. J., & Kredentser, M. S. (2012). Comparative health care use patterns of people with schizophrenia near the end of life: A population-based study in Manitoba, Canada. *Schizophrenia Research, 141*(2–3), 241–246. https://doi.org/10.1016/j.schres.2012.07.028

Curtin, L. (2019). *Killing for profit.* https://www.americannursetoday.com/killing-for-profit/

Fairman, N., & Irwin, S. A. (2013). Palliative care psychiatry: Update on an emerging dimension of psychiatric practice. *Current Psychiatry Reports, 15*(7), 374. https://doi.org/10.1007/s11920-013-0374-3

Ganzini, L., Goy, E. R., Miller, L. L., Harvath, T. A., Jackson, A., & Delorit, M. A. (2003). Nurses' experiences with hospice patients who refuse food and fluids to hasten death. *New England Journal of Medicine, 349*(4), 359–365.

Martins Pereira, S., Fradique, E., & Hernandez-Marrero, P. (2018). End-of-life decision making in palliative care and recommendations of the Council of Europe: Qualitative secondary analysis of interviews and observation field notes. *Journal of Palliative Medicine, 21*(5), 604–615.

Masman, A. D., van Dijk, M., Tibboel, D., Baar, F. P., & Mathôt, R. A. (2015). Medication use during end-of-life care in a palliative care centre. *International Journal of Clinical Pharmacy, 37*(5), 767–775. https://doi.org/10.1007/s11096-015-0094-3

Medical Orders for Life Sustaining Treatment. (2019). *Authority of nurse practitioners under current NYS law.* https://molst.org/ethics-laws/advance-care-planning/authority-of-nurse-practitioners-and-current-nys-law/

Schulte, F. (2017). *Fraud and billing mistakes cost Medicare—and taxpayers—tens of billions last year.* https://khn.org/news/fraud-and-billing-mistakes-cost-medicare-and-taxpayers-tens-of-billions-last-year/

Sorrentino, R. (2014). Performing capacity evaluations: What's expected from your consult. *Current Psychiatry, 13*(1), 41–44.

Taber, J. M., Ellis, E. M., Reblin, M., Ellington, L., & Ferrer, R. A. (2019). Knowledge of and beliefs about palliative care in a nationally-representative US sample. *PLoS One, 14*(8). https://doi.org/10.1371/journal.pone.0219074

Trachsel, M., Irwin, S. A., Biller-Andorno, N., Hoff, P., & Riese, F. (2016). Palliative psychiatry for severe persistent mental illness as a new approach to psychiatry? Definition, scope, benefits, and risks. *BMC Psychiatry, 16*(1), 260. https://doi.org/10.1186/s12888-016-0970-y

World Health Organization (2011). *Palliative care for older people: Better practices.* Retrieved from https://www.euro.who.int/__data/assets/pdf_file/0017/143153/e95052.pdf

World Health Organization. (2018). *Palliative care.* https://www.who.int/news-room/fact-sheets/detail/palliative-care

CHAPTER 15

CARING FOR PATIENTS DURING A PANDEMIC

MARIE SMITH-EAST

LEARNING OBJECTIVE

After reviewing this chapter, practitioners will be able to:

- describe how elderly patients can connect to care during a pandemic such as COVID-19
- explain potential barriers to care for elderly patients during a pandemic
- list examples of approaches that can be used to alleviate exacerbations of psychiatric illness during a pandemic and identify any health disparities
- recommend resources and treatment supports that are available during and after a pandemic

■ INTRODUCTION

During a pandemic such as COVID-19 that creates much uncertainty and rapid changes, supporting elderly patients as well as their families is more integral than ever before. A pandemic is defined as a worldwide spread of an infectious disease (WHO, 2010). Most individuals who are exposed to a crisis such as a pandemic can experience various challenges that can remain in effect even after the pandemic is over. Deaths associated with pandemics, such as with influenza, have been repeatedly reported to affect vulnerable populations, including the elderly and women who are pregnant, at different rates (Morens & Taubenberger, 2018). Specifically regarding the coronavirus (COVID-19) pandemic, eight out of 10 deaths reported in the United States have been adults aged 65 years of age and older (CDC, 2020a).

Although COVID-19 and influenza are both respiratory viral diseases, one of the main differences between the two is the incubation period (with COVID-19 having 14 days before a person would develop symptoms after being exposed, compared to influenza with a 1- to 4-day period) and the rapid spread of the disease (Kaiser Permanente, 2020). With information regarding COVID-19 continually developing, it is essential to be able to efficiently assess, assist, and connect elderly patients to care. Not only should measures be taken to prevent, slow, or stop the spread of the disease during a pandemic, advanced practice nurses must stay up to date on the latest information and guidelines as such approaches are crucial to the manner in which treatment can be provided.

■ BARRIERS AND CONNECTING PATIENTS TO CARE

Foremost, when a pandemic is declared a national emergency, such as with COVID-19 in the United States (Whitehouse.gov, 2020), clinicians must be aware of any changes that can be associated with their ability to connect and provide care to their patients. For example, with national and state emergencies declared during a pandemic, laws can change with regard to the advanced practice nurse's scope of practice in addition to their reimbursement if care has to be provided in a different way. During the COVID-19 pandemic, some states, such as Tennessee, declared a state emergency response to temporarily suspend any waived practice agreement requirements (AANP, 2020) in order to meet needs and address additional challenges that could arise, such as surges in ill patients and staff shortages. Another example is that Medicare has allowed clinicians to provide care via audio-only phone (Medicare.gov, 2020), which is important not just for reimbursement, but will also have an effect on how care is delivered.

Social distancing and the COVID-19 pandemic. As a measure to prevent the rapid spread of COVID-19 among the public, medical guidelines have included social distancing, which is described as physically distancing by providing space at least 6 feet from another individual (CDC, 2020b). Depending on the laws of the country in which the person lives, there may be restrictions to businesses that are open in person or how care is delivered in person, such as the use of masks to reduce spread of the disease or the use of telehealth or telephonic services. Advanced practice nurses must still create an environment that is conducive to a therapeutic relationship through engagement and allowing the patient to feel that the provider is still listening to their thoughts and concerns. Nevertheless, the advanced practice nurse must be prudent in their assessment if using measures that are not in-person, such as video-conferencing and phone use. When providing care to elderly patients, the clinician must be aware of any reluctance that the patient may have to the use of technology and take precautions to keep information shared via phone or technology private and confidential, as well as coordinate with inter-professionals, patient's families, and friends who could assist with connecting via video or smart phone (AMA, 2020).

Barriers to care. During a pandemic, there can be various barriers to care that include communication, psychosocial/ spiritual factors, and access to care. For example, during the COVID-19 pandemic, protocols limited the number of visitors in hospitals and nursing home facilities (Pahuja & Wojcikewych, 2020), which can affect the ability for patients to visit with family, pastors, and even the number of times that a clinician may go into a patient's room. Lack of or limited personal protective equipment during a pandemic such as COVID-19 in addition to the types of services offered, such as annual visits often used for prevention of future illness and elective services can affect provided care (ANA, 2020). Advanced practice nurses can address barriers to care through assessing for the patient's needs and discussing risks versus benefits in treatment, as well as how to implement access to the provider or certain services during the pandemic that outline clear steps. For example, patients may be physically mailed, emailed, or called regarding steps on how their care may be changed and how they will be able to still get care during times of need.

Mitigating disparities. According to the Centers for Disease Control and Prevention (2020c), chronic health system and social disparities exist with increased risk for getting COVID-19 regardless of age among nonHispanic Black individuals, Hispanic/Latinos, and American Indian/Alaskan Natives, who have higher rates of hospitalization or death compared to nonHispanic White individuals. Advanced practice nurses can assist in reducing health disparities by addressing social determinants of health and urging community engagement through working with other sectors in the community (such as transportation, spiritual organizations, education, and businesses) and providing ways to connect to services such as through the clinician's electronic healthcare portal (if available). Advanced practice nurses can also reduce barriers by understanding the needs of the community from their perspective and providing culturally competent care. After the pandemic is over, history regarding emergency response have shown that individuals with mental illness are particularly vulnerable during and after emergencies, and there is need for a plan that embraces practical tools to meet the needs of individuals requiring mental healthcare (WHO, 2019).

■ TREATMENT APPROACHES

SAMHSA (2020) provides considerations for clinicians regarding care during the COVID-19 pandemic, which includes the use of outpatient options (to avoid inpatient care, which could increase risk of infection), the use of telehealth or telephonic services, and staying up to date regarding the latest developments for plan of care during the pandemic. In addition, there are various resources that advanced practice nurses can provide to their patients regarding additional therapeutic support such as crisis text line support (www.crisistextline.org) and online support groups such as the National Alliance on Mental Illness. Proper documentation should reflect each contact with the patient, interprofessionals, including an emphasis on the discussion of a crisis plan. Considerations regarding changes to the home life for elderly individuals should also be made due to the potential for increased social isolation, neglect, and elder abuse (Han & Mosqueda, 2020). Various community-based resources should be utilized including involving local communities to reach patients on a regular basis and offering respite care for caregivers when necessary.

Advanced practice nurses should consider whether changes to medications are necessary (such as increases in medications that could be temporary to address current symptoms like increased anxiety that the patient may have in response to the current pandemic) and whether symptoms can continue to be managed on an outpatient basis. The frequency of visits should also be considered and discussed with the patient, particularly if telephonic services are available, as there may be an option to have more frequent follow-up visits than prior to the pandemic. If telemedicine is used, the clinician should also have a backup telephone number for the patient in case services via video get disconnected. Patient education is also imperative for patients regarding the telemedicine modality prior to the visit, and during the visit, time should be accounted for to address connectivity before the treatment session begins. For patients who may want to decrease their medications during the pandemic, there should be an emphasis with regard to the timing of this during a pandemic. For example, in the event that the patient goes into crisis following a trial reduction of their medication, there could be public restrictions and other implications associated with treatment due to the risk for infection in the hospital setting. Furthermore, continuous assessment and recommendations regarding individual and group therapy, use of community resources, and coping skills are also helpful during this time, as medications may be adjusted.

■ SUMMARY

During and after a pandemic, there are many approaches that advanced practice nurses can take to provide care that considers the social determinants of health and addresses any disparities. Particularly for elderly patients who are 85 years of age and older who are at the greatest risk for severe illness from COVID-19 (CDC, 2020a), staying up to date on laws and medical guidelines is necessary to implement care plans that are current and consider community resources. Such approaches to treatment are critical to the ability of the healthcare team to make adjustments during a time where there may be rapid changes and uncertainty.

CASE 15.1 THE ELDERLY PATIENT USING TELEMEDICINE FOR THE FIRST TIME

An 80-year-old male presents to the advanced practice nurse for a follow-up appointment for mental healthcare services. Typically, the patient comes in person for his appointments; however, due to a state-wide "shelter in place" order, the patient has to see the clinician via telemedicine for the first time. The patient was offered telephonic services as an alternative since he mentioned that he would be using the video platform on his computer for the first time. However, the patient stated that he would rather see the clinician rather than speak via phone. The patient expressed to the clinician that he feels his major depressive disorder is stable on his Lexapro 10 mg, one tablet by mouth every morning, but that he has been having increased anxiety due to watching the news unfold regarding the COVID-19 pandemic. The patient states that he lives alone but that he has a daughter he speaks to once a week.

1. What questions would you consider asking the older adult as part of your assessment?

(continued)

2. During the assessment, his computer freezes and you are not able to see or hear the patient. What would you do next?

3. What are some pharmacological and nonpharmacological approaches that you would do for this patient?

Interprofessional Box

Advanced practice nurses working with other interdisciplinary professions during a pandemic should be aware of their self-care as an essential worker, the impact their self-care can have on the individuals to whom they provide care, and the healthcare system, as such a time can result in psychological distress (APNA, 2020). Advanced practice nurses should continually assess their own physical and mental needs during a pandemic as well to give the best of themselves to their patients, and should be aware of options that are available either in the community or through their place of employment as needs arise (Greenberg et al., 2020). Decisions regarding moral ethics that can affect patients as well as other healthcare professionals can be challenging and the need for additional support through interprofessional collaboration can maximize treatment benefits and resources available for patients. The Centers for Disease Control and Prevention also provides a Clinician On-Call Center that is available 24/7 and offers assistance in answering questions related to diagnostic challenges, clinical management, and infection control measures (services can be reached at: 800-232-4636 or through the CDC website under *Coronavirus Disease 2019 for Healthcare Professionals.*)

Evidence-Based Practice Box

Although pandemics are not new (CDC, 2017), there are ways to slow the spread of illness from a pandemic (CDC, 2020b; WHO, 2020) that should be utilized within communities and healthcare organizations. Measures that can be taken to slow or stop the spread of COVID-19 encompass the engagement of the public, institutions, and governments and involves the use of social distancing, stay-at-home procedures (such as quarantine), wearing masks, assessment and testing, and proper use of standard infection control measures (WHO, 2020). Long-term effects of a pandemic as more information is known over time regarding the disease itself has the potential for significant morbidity, mortality, and social and economic consequences, which will require interventions to mitigate future risk of disruption within communities (Jamison et al., 2017).

REFERENCES

American Association of Nurse Practitioners. (2020). *COVID-19 state emergency response: Temporarily suspended and waived practice agreement requirements.* https://www.aanp.org/advocacy/state/covid-19-state-emergency-response-temporarily-suspended-and-waived-practice-agreement-requirements

American Medical Association. (2020). *How Permanente uses telehealth during the COVID-19 pandemic.* https://www.ama-assn.org/delivering-care/public-health/how-permanente-uses-telehealth-during-covid-19-pandemic

American Nurses Association. (2020). *Adapting standards of care under extreme conditions: Guidance for professionals during disasters.* https://www.nursingworld.org/~4ade15/globalassets/docs/ana/ascec_whitepaper031008final.pdf

American Psychiatric Nurses Association. (2020). *Managing stress and self-care during COVID-19: Information*. https://www.apna.org/i4a/pages/index.cfm?pageid=6685

Centers for Disease Control and Prevention. (2017). *Questions and answers*. https://www.cdc.gov/flu/pandemic-resources/basics/faq.html

Centers for Disease Control and Prevention. (2020a). *Coronavirus disease 2019: Older adults*. https://www.cdc.gov/coronavirus/2019-ncov/need-extra-precautions/older-adults.html

Centers for Disease Control and Prevention. (2020b). *What is social distancing?* https://www.cdc.gov/coronavirus/2019-ncov/prevent-getting-sick/social-distancing.html#:~:text=Social%20distancing%2C%20also%20called,)%20from%20other%20people

Centers for Disease Control and Prevention. (2020c). *Coronavirus disease 2019: Racial and ethnic minority groups*. https://www.cdc.gov/coronavirus/2019-ncov/need-extra-precautions/racial-ethnic-minorities.html

Greenberg, N., Docherty, M., Gnanapragasam, S., & Wessely, S. (2020). Managing mental health challenges faced by healthcare workers during Covid-19 pandemic. *BMJ*, 1–9. https://doi.org/10.1136/bmj.m1211

Han, S. D., & Mosqueda, L. (2020). Elder abuse in the COVID-19 era. *Journal of the American Geriatrics Society*, 1–6. https://doi.org/10.1111/jgs.16496

Jamison, T., Gelband, H., & Horton, S. (2017). *Disease control priorities: Improving health and reducing poverty*. 3rd ed. World Bank Publications.

Kaiser Permanente. (2020). *What makes COVID-19 different?* https://lookinside.kaiserpermanente.org/what-makes-covid-19-different/

Medicare.gov. (2020). *Medicare and coronavirus*. https://www.medicare.gov/medicare-coronavirus

Morens, D. M., & Taubenberger, J. K. (2018). The mother of all pandemics is 100 years old (and going strong). *American*

Journal of Public Health, 108(11), 1449–1454. https://doi.org/10.2105/AJPH.2018.304631

Pahuja, M., & Wojcikewych, D. (2020). Systems barriers to assessment and treatment of COVID-19 positive patients at the end of life. *Journal of Palliative Medicine*, 1–5. https://doi.org/10.1089/jpm.2020.0190

Substance Abuse and Mental Health Services Administration. (2020). *Considerations for the care and treatment of mental and substance use disorders in the COVID-19 epidemic: March 20, 2020.* https://www.samhsa.gov/sites/default/files/considerations-care-treatment-mental-substance-use-disorders-covid19.pdf

Whitehouse.gov. (2020). *Proclamation on declaring a national emergency concerning the novel coronavirus disease (COVID-19) outbreak.* https://www.whitehouse.gov/presidential-actions/proclamation-declaring-national-emergency-concerning-novel-coronavirus-disease-covid-19-outbreak/

World Health Organization. (2010). *What is a pandemic?* https://www.who.int/csr/disease/swineflu/frequently_asked_questions/pandemic/en/

World Health Organization. (2019). *Mental health in emergencies.* https://www.who.int/news-room/fact-sheets/detail/mental-health-in-emergencies

World Health Organization. (2020). *Coronavirus disease 2019 situation report.* https://www.who.int/docs/default-source/coronaviruse/situation-reports/20200401-sitrep-72-covid-19.pdf?sfvrsn=3dd8971b_2

Index

Printed in the United States
by Baker & Taylor Publisher Services

Printed in the United States
by Baker & Taylor Publisher Services